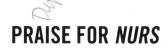

PRAISE FOR *NURS*

"This wonderfully rich and highly relev *provement initiatives in a variety of healthcare settings. The book is filled with practical and effective strategies for staff engagement, from the first steps in defining a problem through sustaining meaningful change. Sample tools, communications to team members, and methods for inspiring enjoyment while doing the work are useful for all teams getting started on their improvement journey."*

–Frances J. Damian, MS, RN, NEA-BC
Director of Nursing/Patient Services
Emergency Services, Boston Children's Hospital

"A compelling read for all healthcare providers. The authors share their ambitious vision, associated concepts, and real-life examples of their value-creation journey on the frontlines of healthcare delivery. Everything is provided, including their framework and actual templates. No stone goes unturned in addressing the necessary cultural and operational aspects of this transformational project. After reading this book, executives and clinical nurses will better see the value proposition through each other's eyes."

–Christopher D. Masotti, CPA, MBA
Vice Dean of Finance and Operations
Perelman School of Medicine, University of Pennsylvania

"The authors use an innovative strategy to engage clinical nurses in financial savings. The transformational CHOP framework empowers nurses with the mind-set, culture, structure, and process to continuously remove clinical supply waste. The success factors and improvement tools shared are best practice models for replication in any healthcare setting. Nursing-Led Savings *will ignite nurses with invaluable skills to elevate quality while simultaneously reducing cost—our collective mandate for affordable healthcare!"*

–Nancy Dunn, MS, RN
Clinical Excellence Coordinator, Salem Health

"*This book is a must-read for every healthcare executive and anyone else interested in improving the healthcare value proposition by reducing nonlabor expenses. Through highlighting their methods and successes at Children's Hospital of Philadelphia, the authors produced a practical, easy-to-read, and informative quality improvement primer. No matter where you are on your personal understanding of improvement science and change management, you will learn something new from this book.*"

–Rustin B. Morse, MD, MMM
SVP, Quality and Safety
Chief Quality Officer
Interim Chief Clinical Officer
Children's Health System of Texas

"*This book is the product of the perfect blend of leadership from all perspectives working together to make a difference. The authors put together a wonderful blueprint that combines leadership, quality, empowerment, and fiscal responsibility to inspire others to action. By working through failures, opportunities, research, and achievements, the CHOP model sets the stage for success. A must-read for all nurses and a great resource to share with other healthcare professionals!*"

–AnnMarie Papa, DNP, RN, CEN, NE-BC, FAEN, FAAN
Vice President & Chief Nursing Officer
Einstein Medical Center Montgomery

"Nursing-Led Savings *is an imaginative approach to cost savings in an ever-changing healthcare industry. It's a unique look at initiating those savings at the bedside and how to engage staff in the process. I highly recommend this book for all levels of hospital personnel.*"

–Kellie C. Dyer, MBA
Director, Supply Chain
Valley Children's Healthcare

"It makes sense to have nurses lead savings initiatives within their hospitals. This is not just about putting nurses on another committee and telling them to go save money. It is an innovative approach that combines real-world nursing experience with the latest savings strategies in the healthcare world."

–Robert Yokl
Senior Vice President of Operations
SVAH Solutions

Nursing-Led Savings

The Children's Hospital of Philadelphia guide to cost-saving solutions, bedside financial stewardship, and improved efficiency in care-delivery systems

Paula Agosto, MHA, RN
Megan Bernstein, BSN, RN, CPN, CCRN
Cheryl Gebeline-Myers, MS
Jackie Noll, MSN, RN, CEN
Jessica Steck, BSN, RN, CPN

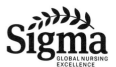

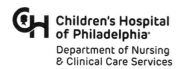
Children's Hospital of Philadelphia
Department of Nursing & Clinical Care Services

The Sigma Theta Tau International Honor Society of Nursing (Sigma) is a nonprofit organization whose mission is advancing world health and celebrating nursing excellence in scholarship, leadership, and service. Founded in 1922, Sigma has more than 135,000 active members in over 90 countries and territories. Members include practicing nurses, instructors, researchers, policymakers, entrepreneurs, and others. Sigma's more than 530 chapters are located at more than 700 institutions of higher education throughout Armenia, Australia, Botswana, Brazil, Canada, Colombia, England, Ghana, Hong Kong, Ireland, Jamaica, Japan, Jordan, Kenya, Lebanon, Malawi, Mexico, the Netherlands, Nigeria, Pakistan, Philippines, Portugal, Puerto Rico, Singapore, South Africa, South Korea, Swaziland, Sweden, Taiwan, Tanzania, Thailand, the United States, and Wales. Learn more at www.sigmanursing.org.

Sigma Theta Tau International
550 West North Street
Indianapolis, IN, USA 46202

To order additional books, buy in bulk, or order for corporate use, contact Sigma Marketplace at 888.654.4968 (US and Canada) or +1.317.634.8171 (outside US and Canada).

To request a review copy for course adoption, email solutions@sigmamarketplace.org or call 888.654.4968 (US and Canada) or +1.317.634.8171 (outside US and Canada).

To request author information, or for speaker or other media requests, contact Sigma Marketing at 888.634.7575 (US and Canada) or +1.317.634.8171 (outside US and Canada).

ISBN: 9781948057165
EPUB ISBN: 9781948057172
PDF ISBN: 9781948057189
MOBI ISBN: 9781948057196

Library of Congress Cataloging-in-Publication data

Names: Agosto, Paula, author. | Bernstein, Megan, 1985- author. |
  Gebeline-Myers, Cheryl, 1979- author. | Noll, Jackie, author. | Steck,
  Jessica, author. | Sigma Theta Tau International, publisher.
Title: Nursing-led savings : the Children's Hospital of Philadelphia guide
  to cost-saving solutions, bedside financial stewardship, and improved
  efficiency in care-delivery systems / Paula Agosto, Megan Bernstein,
  Cheryl Gebeline-Myers, Jackie Noll, Jessica Steck.
Description: Indianapolis : Sigma Theta Tau International, [2020] | Includes
  bibliographical references and index.
Identifiers: LCCN 2019021240| ISBN 9781948057165 | ISBN
9781948057196 (mobi)
  | ISBN 9781948057189 (pdf) | ISBN 9781948057172 (epub)
Subjects: | MESH: Economics, Nursing | Cost Savings--methods | Shared
  Governance, Nursing | Efficiency, Organizational--economics
Classification: LCC RT86.7 | NLM WY 77 | DDC 610.73068/1--dc23 LC
record available at https://lccn.loc.gov/2019021240

First Printing, 2019

Publisher: Dustin Sullivan
Acquisitions Editor: Emily Hatch
Publications Specialist: Todd Lothery
Cover Designer: Rebecca Batchelor
Interior Design/Page Layout:
Rebecca Batchelor

Managing Editor: Carla Hall
Development and Project Editor:
Rebecca Senninger
Copy Editor: Erin Geile
Proofreader: Gill Editorial Services
Indexer: Joy Dean Lee

DEDICATION

To the clinical bedside nurses who tried something new and succeeded. You transformed a culture and continue to lead this every day.

ACKNOWLEDGMENTS

We would like to point out first and foremost that this work took a tremendous team effort and includes numerous colleagues across the Children's Hospital of Philadelphia enterprise. In reality, we could acknowledge almost every employee—every nurse, every improvement professional, every leader—as financial stewardship is everyone's work. Our workforce embraced the culture change, and for this, we are grateful. There are a few people whose remarkable contributions framed the work and fueled success. These folks are the unsung heroes, and they include Debra Geiger, Eric Branning, Tyshawn Toney, Bob Yokl, Alice Harrington, Maggie McGrath, Mary Jo Gumbel, Peter Schemm, Elaine Gallagher, the CHOPtimize team members, Elvin Vega, Andy Parshall, and Tom Todorow. We need them to rest up, as this work is never done!

Of course, we would be remiss not to thank our families for their endless support in the very hard work we do every day and their understanding of how much we truly love what we do.

ABOUT THE AUTHORS

Paula Agosto, MHA, RN, is the Chief Nurse Officer at Children's Hospital of Philadelphia. Agosto started her career at CHOP as a staff nurse in the Pediatric Intensive Care Unit (PICU) in 1985. Since 1996, she has assumed progressively responsible leadership roles, including Nurse Manager of the PICU; Director of Critical Care, Transport, and Emergency Nursing; and Assistant Vice President of Critical Care, Respiratory and Neuro-Diagnostic services. In addition to her extensive leadership experience, Agosto has led a number of successful cross-organizational improvement and operating plan initiatives. Having earned her nursing degree from Villanova University and a master of health administration from Saint Joseph's University, she has written for numerous pediatric textbooks and manuals and has given presentations around the country on pediatric nursing topics. Agosto is responsible for advancing nursing and respiratory practice and leading advancements in nursing research while supporting CHOP's commitment to exceptional patient care.

Megan Bernstein, BSN, RN, CPN, CCRN, is a Clinical Nurse Expert in the Pediatric Intensive Care Unit (PICU) at CHOP, where she has been a nurse since 2007. She started her nursing career in the Progressive Care Unit at CHOP and transitioned to the PICU after two years, where she has progressed to a leadership role. With her certification in pediatric and critical care nursing, Bernstein continues to practice bedside nursing in the PICU. She was the acting Department Chair for the Supporting Practice and Management (SPM) Council for Nursing Shared Governance at CHOP, where she helped to facilitate and embed the CHOPtimize initiative at the bedside level. She has presented her work at national and international nursing and healthcare conferences.

Cheryl Gebeline-Myers, MS, is the Senior Director of Clinical Services and Programs in the Office of Safety & Medical Operations at CHOP. She has a 20-year record of successful contributions in research, quality, safety, and process improvement in various sectors of the healthcare industry. This includes training frontline staff and healthcare leaders in the application of structured improvement methodologies. Holding a master's degree in healthcare quality from George Washington University School of Medicine and Health Sciences, Gebeline-Myers has led poster and platform presentations and interactive workshops across numerous national and international conferences on topics spanning quality and patient safety, financial stewardship, resident education, and Lean in healthcare. She has authored several peer-reviewed publications and book chapters and serves as adjunct faculty at Thomas Jefferson University. She is a coinventor of a newly designed and licensed product to protect peripheral IVs in patients.

Jackie Noll, MSN, RN, CEN, is a Senior Director of Nursing at CHOP. She earned a BSN degree from Thomas Jefferson University and an MSN degree in leadership and health system management from Drexel University. Noll's operational scope within the Department of Nursing includes the emergency department (ED), the ED Extended Care Unit, Sedation/Radiology, Interventional Radiology, and Vascular Access Services. Having begun her career in intensive care as a clinical staff RN, Noll has over 30 years of experience in nursing, including years in leadership roles. She enjoys strategic start-up planning and implementation, and she helped develop the CHOP Home Care department and Urgent Care sites. She also led enterprise plan initiative teams in workforce productivity, harm prevention, improving patient experience, and nonlabor cost reduction. She is the clinical co-chair of the Value Analysis Committee, known as CHOPtimize, focused on maximizing value in patient care supplies. Passionate about developing and mentoring nurses to lead at all levels in the organization, Noll speaks nationally on clinical and leadership topics, and she is published in patient safety walk rounds.

Jessica Steck, BSN, RN, CPN, is a Clinical Nurse in the After Hours Program for CHOP. With a certification in pediatric nursing, she was the Shared Governance unit-based representative for her unit and was instrumental in championing and leading CHOPtimize work at the bedside. Steck has presented her work on nursing engagement in nonlabor expense reduction at national and international healthcare conferences.

TABLE OF CONTENTS

3 ESTABLISHING THE "WHO": ENLISTING THE BEDSIDE NURSES 58

4 IMPROVEMENT METHODOLOGY: TRANSLATING THE "HOW" 78

5 NURSING-LED SAVINGS IN ACTION: A BEDSIDE NURSE'S PERSPECTIVE AND STORY 106

FOREWORD

If you want to get something done, ask a nurse. If you want something done right, ask a nurse. That's what we did at Children's Hospital of Philadelphia (CHOP): We asked our nurses to help us become more responsible stewards of our resources. We asked them to help us find ways to cut costs and become more efficient. And they delivered, offering innovative and effective ideas that we are now putting into practice in our hospital and across our Care Network. We have reduced the cost of care, and our patient-families are seeing the benefits because we are able to pass some of these savings on to them.

At CHOP, we spend a lot of time focused on scenario planning, and finances are always an important part of these discussions. I believe that the one thing all hospitals and healthcare organizations can do to ensure their success in any future scenario is to lower costs. Yet very few know how to do this—and an even smaller group have asked nurses to lead the charge.

I am proud that CHOP is part of this group, and I am thrilled that our nursing team has written this book to share their insights and expertise. Whether you are a clinical frontline staff or an executive leader—I started at CHOP as a nurse in 1983, so I am familiar with both roles—this book will help you empower your teams to create change. Because nurses are on the front lines of patient care, they have the best ideas for improving how hospitals work. They simply need a practical how-to guide like this one to help them put their ideas into action.

–Madeline Bell
President and CEO
Children's Hospital of Philadelphia

INTRODUCTION

"Unless someone like you cares a whole awful lot,
nothing is going to get better. It's not."
–Dr. Seuss

We would like to formally welcome you to our book. Yes, we
started with a Dr. Seuss quote. We can't help ourselves—we
work at a children's hospital after all. The quote rings true,
though. You have begun reading this book because you
are interested in making a positive change for your organization. This book shares an organizational journey at
Children's Hospital of Philadelphia—a journey originating
out of necessity but, most importantly, out of responsibility
to the mission and patients we serve as well as the broader
healthcare landscape. We highlight a framework for leveraging a Nursing Shared Governance model and a structured
improvement methodology for staff to lead cost-reduction
efforts at the bedside. This how-to guide will walk organizational leaders at all levels through the development and
implementation of a robust cost-saving strategy focusing
directly on eliminating waste and streamlining processes
in everyday clinical work. We will also provide you with
the toolkit to do it. This strategy involves prioritization of
nonlabor expense reduction at the senior leadership levels,
engaging Nursing Shared Governance councils in oversight
and implementation of the work, educating frontline staff on
the importance of financial stewardship, and using a structured approach to improvement methodology to execute the
cost-saving efforts at the bedside.

In light of the increasing costs associated with healthcare, we have an obligation as healthcare professionals to decrease costs by reducing waste and overall inefficiencies. The changing climate in healthcare reform poses uncertainty for hospitals and health systems. Planning for the unexpected is necessary to ensure continued mission stewardship for these organizations. A typical business approach to cost savings is to focus on your most costly expense—in most instances, human capital. However, with increasing capacity demands for healthcare providers, the impact of cutting labor expenses alone are substantial—it can result in a loss of high-quality, safe care for patients. This book provides an alternate strategy for hospital leaders to deploy as part of their cost-reduction efforts—a focus on nonlabor expense reduction and methods for engaging your frontline care providers in driving the cost-saving solutions.

You may be at the beginning stages of financial stewardship in your organization or well along in your cost-saving journey and looking to learn more about better engaging frontline nursing. In this book, you will hear from a variety of different "voices" and perspectives—from senior executive leadership, senior nursing leaders, a former Nursing Shared Governance chair, process improvement professionals, and of course, bedside nurses. Each will share the nursing-led savings journey through their own lens, providing you, the reader, with an in-depth understanding of what it means to lead this work across all levels. These voices and perspectives vary, which is the exact flavor we are looking to deliver.

Chapter 1 explains why embedding financial stewardship work is an imperative for organizations and how to engage staff by improving financial awareness at all levels.

Chapter 2 describes how to build your organizational structures to support the enterprise improvement work needed to achieve organizational goals in cost reduction.

Chapter 3 discusses strategies to engage bedside nurses in the work and the importance of finding a common language when executives and frontline staff work together.

Chapter 4 provides an approach to leveraging a structured improvement framework that effectively supports bedside nurses in leading meaningful change.

Chapter 5 highlights the work of the frontline nurse and how her day-to-day decisions affect the financial bottom line.

Chapter 6 summarizes the themes of our work and how our efforts continue to evolve with new generations of team members.

Finally, the appendix presents a key driver diagram for the overarching approach to engaging nurses in leading cost-saving efforts. A *key driver diagram* is essentially a road map of what must go right in order to meet your global aim. Whenever we felt stuck, we would revisit this diagram to show how far we had come and to highlight the next step in the journey. This is the road map we used, but we believe it can be easily translated to other organizations and projects.

We hope you will learn from our journey, be inspired to make change, and achieve your own desired outcomes. Along your own journey, you have an opportunity to share your success stories locally, but we also hope you can share your experiences with us. We strive to achieve continued outcomes in this work and want to hear from you on lessons learned and best practices. Indeed, nurses add incredible value by eliminating waste and improving efficiency in our care-delivery systems. Ultimately, we want you to be the catalyst in your organization to use a similar approach and make a difference for your patients and your mission. Our patients count on us for excellence in both healthcare and value. Nurses, please continue to embrace your role as financial stewards, and you will create a better future for all.

"If we want things to stay as they are, things will have to change."
–Giuseppe Tomasi di Lampedusa

1

FINANCIAL STEWARDSHIP: FRAMING THE "WHY"

Paula Agosto, MHA, RN, Senior Vice President and Chief Nurse Officer; Jackie Noll, MSN, RN, CEN, Senior Director of Nursing

WORDS &
CONCEPTS TO LEARN

Financial margin

*Financial
stewardship*

Healthcare reform

Mission sustainability

Payer mix

Payer mix shifts

Shared Governance

*Shared Governance departmental and
unit-based councils*

Value

Healthcare systems and healthcare delivery affect every nurse. At any given time, nurses are consumers or providers of healthcare—or both. They expect and demand high value for themselves and their patients. Indeed, every nurse has a responsibility to use or provide healthcare resources wisely and efficiently to create a high-value experience.

The evolving healthcare system is experiencing high costs of services and supplies, which are outpacing a consumer's ability to afford care. Those working in the healthcare system can be overwhelmed when strategizing how to best manage the complexities of the system, rising patient acuity, and increasing demand, while keeping costs down and maximizing efficiencies.

HEALTHCARE LANDSCAPE: THE EVOLVING UNCERTAINTY

To ignite the interests of your organization's staff to buy into the vision of improving your own systems, start by sharing the troubling current state of healthcare spending. The staggering high costs in healthcare create a big threat to patient care-delivery models in the United States. You need to change the way you work as part of the solution to control costs. *All nurses can act locally to impact globally, and it all starts with education and transparency.*

Population Impacts

Healthcare costs in the United States are consistently a top concern for Americans (Jones & Reinhart, 2018), and there is no simple solution to mitigate these costs. Healthcare spending reached 17.9% of the gross domestic product in 2016, and healthcare spending is projected to grow at 5.5% from 2017 to 2026 (Centers for Medicare and Medicaid Services [CMS], Office of the Actuary, National Health Statistics Group, 2018). In fact, although US utilization rates are largely similar to those in other nations, the US spends approximately twice as much as other high-income countries on medical care (Papanicolas, Woskie, & Jha, 2018). Papanicolas et al. (2018) note the prices of labor and goods, as well as administrative costs, stand out as the major differences from other high-income countries.

Individual Impacts

Staff also are sensitive to consumer-level impacts. CMS shares the increasing number of high-deductible policies that are greatly impacting people, and the trend is concerning (CMS, 2018). In fact, out-of-pocket expenditure is approximately 11% of the national health expenditure (CMS, 2018). Patients, families, and even staff are feeling the burden of rising healthcare costs. Staff feel the financial stressors of their patients, as well as recognize them as direct consumers of healthcare.

Clearly, the future of healthcare spending needs practical and realistic reform; nurses, along with their interdisciplinary colleagues, are poised to drive change in lowering costs. Nurses are vital as financial stewards of healthcare resources to ensure a strong and accessible healthcare-delivery model for the future. Removing inefficiencies and waste will lower the overall product and system costs.

A talented workforce has influence here! Specifically, your nursing workforce is educated to be a driving force in innovation and excellence (American Association of Colleges of Nursing, 2019). Nurses can use their strengths in building multidisciplinary partnerships to influence change in your organizations. They are prepared to be catalysts in helping to lower healthcare costs.

MISSION SUSTAINABILITY: ESTABLISHING AN ORGANIZATIONAL PRIORITY

Financial stewardship is the careful and responsible management of something precious entrusted to your care. In the case of healthcare resources, financial stewardship gives access to affordable healthcare, decreases the stress on healthcare institutions to cut back important services, and allows for resources needed for other activities to be available to improve the health of a population.

Mission sustainability is a concept others need to understand in your financial stewardship work. The overall organizational mission informs the vision and values. Healthcare organizations often create their mission, vision, and values as guiding principles for decision-making and strategy. For instance, an organization may define its mission as providing excellent patient care, advancing research, and educating staff. This mission signals the employees to create structures and processes supporting patient care, research, and education. Without a solid financial foundation, the organization and its mission are at great risk. The organization may need to reduce services or even close. Therefore, it is crucial to remind your staff of your organizational mission and to share the importance of keeping the organization's financial well-being in mind, so the mission can continue.

A *financial margin* in a healthcare system is the difference between the total costs the organization needs to provide patient care services and the total net revenue or reimbursement for those services. A positive margin indicates profits; a negative margin indicates financial loss. Maintaining a positive profit margin is critical to mission sustainability.

Healthcare executives are constantly challenged to respond to the evolving healthcare environment. Executive leaders and their executive boards seek to lower expenditures, while still achieving high-quality outcomes. The staff at large need to embrace the concept that financial margins support the organizational mission.

NOTE

Healthcare costs continue to escalate while reimbursement continues to drop. Everyone in your organization needs to be a good financial steward of your resources. It is your responsibility to make sure your care is not only the highest quality, but also a value to your patients and families.

A big step in making the journey to mission sustainability is to educate staff on current organizational margins and the multitude of outside forces affecting them. Staff need to know about healthcare reform, the changing payer mix, and how any shift in the payer mix affects the bottom line. Sharing information about the financial well-being of the organization is pivotal in helping the employees understand why executives are looking to improve efficiencies and lower costs. Financial awareness education occurs first in the Shared Governance councils; they, in turn, can then further share the content at the unit level. Chapter 3 has more information about Shared Governance. Financial transparency helps unite efforts and understanding across all levels of the organization.

HEALTHCARE FINANCIAL TERMS

Healthcare reform: Governmental legislation to improve access to healthcare for everyone.

Payer mix: Healthcare terminology for the percentage of revenue coming from private insurance versus government insurance versus self-paying individuals.

Payer mix shifts: The payer mix is important because Medicare and Medicaid typically pay hospitals less than what it costs to treat patients. Hospitals can track and trend payer mix changes to forecast their profit margins.

Shared Governance: Provides a mechanism for nurses to inform decisions that improve patient care and the work environment. Shared Governance fosters an environment of participation, accountability, empowerment, and respect that strengthens and improves the delivery of evidence-based, patient-centered care.

Shared Governance departmental and unit-based councils: These are the forums for decision-making in the nursing department. The departmental council is hospital-wide and shares work across the organization. The unit-based council engages local staff to participate in the department initiatives and raise issues and suggestions to the departmental council. These councils retain the responsibility and accountability for the process and outcome of all issues related to professional practice, research, quality improvement, education, and leadership.

Additionally, it is important to not mislead staff into thinking executives are strictly approaching the strategy to reduce costs through a financial perspective alone. Indeed, organizational strategy is aimed at driving for *value,* a product of quality divided by cost (Value = Quality/Cost). Therefore, to achieve high value and high quality, you must control costs. At times, employees may perceive the mission to lower costs will result in lowering quality of care. Employees often say "don't give me a cheaper product" when they hear the need to lower costs. Take the time to identify these concerns and address them. Employees raise concerns if a cheaper product reduces the quality, because the value to the patient is then also reduced. On the other hand, if a product's quality improves while the cost is reduced, employees' support increases due to the value added to the patient's care. Sharing the value equation and providing examples of how the value equation works in your organization is a wise step in embedding an organization's cost-reduction priority.

Commit to using an approach to promote and endorse the importance of the value equation being the guiding principle for your financial stewardship work. Make sure leaders at all levels in your organization understand the concept and embrace the approach. Identify or create opportunities to share examples with both leaders and staff often. You can describe examples of value in action at departmental or small group meetings, in newsletters, via posters, and in one-to-one interactions. Providing real examples of this equation in action helps embed it into your culture. We talk about an example that changed our culture in Chapter 5.

 NOTE

Nonlabor cost reduction is something you need to become nimble with in healthcare for mission sustainability. Be transparent about your hospital's financial position, describe national trends, tell stories of patient deductibles, and relate the concepts to their life experiences. Look for the early adopters, and support their ideas.

TRANSLATING FINANCIAL STEWARDSHIP AT THE BEDSIDE: ENGAGING THE MIND AND HEART

To maximize the potential of staff participation, it is important to understand what motivates employees. It is equally important to understand who composes your workforce. The majority of staff represent two generations: Generation X and millennials. Each generation has its unique traits:

- **Generation X** are described by Gentry, Griggs, Deal, Mondore, and Cox in 2011 as "individualistic, risk-tolerant, self-reliant, entrepreneurial, comfortable with diversity, and valuing work life balance" (p. 41). In this specific work, Generation X can help seek alternatives to the status quo.

- **Millennials,** as described by Howe and Strauss in 2000, are overachievers and are accountable for their actions. They are able to multitask and improvise when needed. Millennials provide a strong sense of commitment to create change for the greater good.

Creating an approach where all generations feel valued is a key to the success of any program, and certainly was the key to success for Children's Hospital of Philadelphia (CHOP).

Strong financial stewardship requires not only a focus on individual contributions, but also effective teamwork. In addition to generational differences, some colleagues will be more resistant to change than others. As you lead through change, remember to respect the needs and timelines each adopter brings to the process.

According to Everett Rogers (Agency for Clinical Innovation, 2015), there are five types of change management adopters:

- **Innovators:** First to adopt change and are your risk takers

- **Early adopters:** Likely includes those who offer opinions and accept change early

- **Early majority:** Take longer to adopt new ideas and not often opinion leaders

- **Late majority:** Adopt an innovation after the average member adopts and approach change with skepticism

- **Laggards:** The last group to change and are change-averse

For those resisting change, you need to help them see how continued change is needed to advance care delivery each day. Creating a fund of knowledge and understanding for all (regarding the benefits of reducing costs and waste throughout the system) builds a sound foundation on which to build future work. Numerous lessons can be shared about overall healthcare spending trends and their impact on the community, healthcare organizations, and, most importantly, patients and staff. Scan for current examples both internal and external to your organization. Follow local and national news along with briefings from your professional journals for insight into healthcare spending issues and impacts.

We previously noted how rising healthcare costs have gained national attention, yet it can be a challenge to engage those in healthcare delivery in making improvements. Some organizations try to approach the challenge of lowering costs by setting executive-level expectations and directives. While this imperative may make sense at the highest levels in organizations, the fundamental changes do not consistently translate to the staff who are directly interfacing with patients and the resources available. It is the responsibility of formal or informal leaders to create the desire and emotional energy to make and sustain improvements.

While this work began at CHOP, staff voiced a clear disconnect between the intention to reduce costs and what they experience in practice. In general, staff did not see the reason for change. They saw financial security and a developing healthcare system as a sign of financial health for the organization. Therefore, there was a lack of urgency or "a burning platform" for cost reduction and resource management in the eyes of the staff.

The critical step in making improvements in a healthcare system is engaging staff. As is covered in Chapter 3, we approached the work of financial stewardship by leveraging the talents and experiences of frontline staff. We used the Shared Governance council to connect with frontline staff who are in the best position to see and influence direct care delivery. The staff are the foundations of financial stewardship.

Improving Financial Awareness

"I am a clinical nurse" is what echoes in the minds and hearts of nurses when asked about how to reduce expenses in their care delivery. Nurses receive undergraduate degrees in science, not business. When executives discuss the business of healthcare with staff, nurses often express how foreign and uncomfortable they feel discussing costs and using the financial terminology.

The first strategy is to push through the resistance from staff's lack of understanding. Make your education and awareness campaign on the business of healthcare a priority. Take the time to educate your staff.

Recognizing the goal of creating financial stewardship begins with building business capabilities in the clinical staff; an education and awareness campaign is a critically important first step. The staff who directly care for patients need to understand:

- The business environment of the healthcare organization
- What is happening in the nation, in the region, and in the immediate community

- Budget concepts, an understanding of scale and how it relates to purchasing, population growth, the overview details of the organizational annual financials, and the vision of executive leadership and the institution's board of trustees

The time and training with the Nursing Shared Governance staff and clinical leaders in your organization are an investment with a high-yield result.

Conveying Relatable Concepts

Begin all education by making the finance concepts relatable. Describing a basic home budget allows you to connect the hospital budgeting concepts to the lives of your staff. Teach about expenses versus revenues and the reason for a budget, but you do not need to stop there. Share the greater organizational balance sheet. Explain what profit margins are and how healthy margins affect your ratings for borrowing money. Keep explanations simple while explaining the organization's Standard & Poor's or Moody's rating. People understand these rating concepts if they can relate this scoring to their lives. For instance, remind staff if they have lower debt and higher income, they can get lower interest rates for buying a home or a car. Share how an organization's sustainability is related to keeping these financial balance sheets healthy and ensuring ratings are in the best position possible.

> ## FINANCIAL RATINGS
>
> A Standard & Poor's or a Moody's financial rating gives an organization a letter grade to reflect its financial health. The best is "AAA." This rating means it is highly likely that the borrower will repay its debt. The worst is "D," which means the issuer has already defaulted.

Discovering Inefficiencies

The one area staff are very comfortable speaking about is waste. This is where you can capitalize on their insights and couple those insights with their updated understanding of finances. Staff can easily identify processes and products in their day-to-day work that seem broken. Ask them to think about:

- What they throw away when they open prepackaged kits

- How often they walk too far for supplies that could be located nearby

- How often they use supplies for something the manufacturer does not intend

- What products continually fail

Staff live with inefficiencies and see waste every day. To make the concept of waste relatable, share examples of waste they could experience in their everyday lives.

Show staff the impact of overstocked rooms with supplies and linens that cannot be used again for other patients, or perhaps what happens when they open a dressing kit and throw away one of the supplies because it is not exactly what they need. All this waste needs to be defined, and who better to do this than the staff? It is empowering to know that there are steps each of them can take to lower the cost of care.

In Chapter 4, we talk about creating process maps where staff walk through the work steps and identify inefficiencies. Process maps are the building blocks for the work ahead in reducing the cost of care.

INCLUDING A STORY/PERSONAL PERSPECTIVE

Sharing the "why" behind the organizational initiative to reduce the cost of care is critical. Build staff capabilities to understand the external and internal forces affecting care delivery and costs. Embrace transparency with the staff, because they are the ones who have the closest view of what is right and what is broken in the institution's system. The strategy to leverage Nursing Shared Governance and embrace a bottom-up approach to this work puts the responsibility in the hands of the right people—nurses who are delivering care directly.

This work marks the beginning of a journey, and many followers will be needed along the way. Leverage executives to help share the vision. Invite the Chief Nursing Officer (CNO), Chief Financial Officer (CFO), and Vice President of Supply Chain Management to attend a Shared Governance meeting. Ask each executive to deliver a 60-second elevator speech on the need for an enterprise initiative to reduce costs.

Each executive leader will have a brief and inspiring message that can be repeated to others. For example, the CHOP CFO challenged us to think about any process or product that seemed to be ineffective or inefficient in our day-to-day work. He shared that saving one dollar a day per person in an organization with 11,000 people could save over $4 million per year. The CNO shared the message of financial stewardship and the critical role nurses fulfill in making a difference, and she challenged us to take action. Finally, the VP of Supply Chain Management explained the resources and improvement methodologies that we would be using to make an impact. She shared the exact organizational goals over the next three years and encouraged us to challenge the norm. The executive leaders explained they would return in a year to hear the elevator speeches from the representatives in the room about their ideas, their successes, and even their failures.

The elevator speech exercise brought two groups together who had the same mission but often were not in the same room working together. The concise messages could easily be recalled and shared among staff not present at all organizational levels. The support from the top leaders was palpable, along with the energy created in the room.

📁 NOTE

Make the beginnings memorable, and infuse energy and engagement as the "why" is explained. Comfort in doing something different should be encouraged. Adding humor is a helpful adjunct. What will best resonate with these teams is how the institution's administrative and executive leaders made them feel; most importantly, make them feel like partners who are invaluable in this work.

Successfully managing the "why" fosters the foundation needed to get to the "how." Establishing an engaging platform for change allows staff to embrace the work with a sense of purpose, creating clear goals for success. The energy created at this phase opens the door to creative thinking, detailed problem-solving, and, most importantly, personal accountability for initiating and sustaining change. This first crucial step sets the course for success as the work begins.

REFERENCES

Agency for Clinical Innovation. (2015). *Change management theories and models – Everett Rogers.* Retrieved from https://www.aci. health.nsw.gov.au/__data/assets/pdf_file/0010/298756/Change_ Management_Theories_and_Models_Everett_Rogers.pdf

American Association of Colleges of Nursing. (2019). Nursing education programs. Retrieved from https://www.aacnnursing.org/Nursing-Education

Centers for Medicare and Medicaid Services. (2018). *NHE fact sheet.* Retrieved from https://www.cms.gov/Research-Statistics-Data-and-Systems/Statistics-Trends-and-Reports/NationalHealthExpendData/ NHE-Fact-Sheet.html

Centers for Medicare and Medicaid Services, Office of the Actuary, National Health Statistics Group. (2018). *National health expenditure projections 2017–26: Major findings.* Retrieved from https://www.cms. gov/Research-Statistics-Data-and-Systems/Statistics-Trends-and-Reports/NationalHealthExpendData/Downloads/NHEProjSlides. pdf

Gentry, W. A., Griggs, T. L., Deal, J. J., Mondore, S. P., & Cox, B. D. (2011). A comparison of generational differences in endorsement of leadership practices with actual leadership skill level. *Consulting Psychology Journal: Practice and Research, 63*(1), 39–49. http://dx.doi. org/10.1037/a0023015

Howe, N., & Strauss, W. (2000). *Millennials rising: The next great generation.* New York, NY: Vintage Books.

Jones, J. M., & Reinhart, R. J. (2018, November 28). Americans remain dissatisfied with healthcare costs. *Gallup.* Retrieved from https:// news.gallup.com/poll/245054/americans-remain-dissatisfied-health-care-costs.aspx

Papanicolas, I., Woskie, L. R., & Jha, A. K. (2018). Health care spending in the United States and other high-income countries. *JAMA, 319*(10), 1024–1039. doi: 10.1001/jama.2018.1150

"The first step to getting anywhere is deciding you're no longer willing to stay where you are."
–Anonymous

2

BUILDING THE ORGANIZATIONAL STRUCTURE: DESIGNING THE "WHAT"

Amy Gallagher, MHA, PharmD, RPh, AVP Operations; Jackie Noll, MSN, RN, Senior Director of Nursing; Joni Rittler, VP Supply Chain Management

WORDS &
CONCEPTS TO LEARN

Action plan

*Governance
structure*

Multidisciplinary teams

Everyone involved in healthcare in the past few decades knows that change is inevitable and continual. However, even experienced executives may cringe when faced with reducing expenses. The goal for Children's Hospital of Philadelphia (CHOP) in 2012 was to cut $45 million. An intimidating number! But one that was necessary to mitigate any impact of impending reimbursement changes. For a pediatric hospital, changes to Medicaid or to the Children's Health Insurance Program can have dramatic impacts. CHOP wanted to be prepared for an uncertain future.

No matter what your budget is or the amount that you need to reduce, your hospital can follow the same strategy.

TAKING ON THE CHALLENGE OF REDUCING EXPENSES

For CHOP, nonlabor expenses are the second largest expense, exceeded only by labor and benefits. Nonlabor expenses include all the costs for supplies, equipment, and services. For a hospital, nonlabor expense hits a broad range of categories, including medical and office supplies, medical and office equipment, computers and technology, and major capital equipment (costing millions of dollars). Additionally, service contracts include preventative maintenance for equipment and systems, landscaping, rotary and ambulatory services, and consulting, to name just a few.

TALES FROM THE FRONT LINE

My name is Joni Rittler, and as the Vice President of Supply Chain Management, it is my role to provide guidance and strategies to manage nonlabor expenses. The expense reduction initiative was targeted as a project on CHOP's enterprise plan for fiscal year 2012, and I was the executive sponsor of the initiative. From my past experience, I knew we had to involve many people from across the organization to be successful in this effort. Also, I wanted the project to be fun and for everyone at CHOP to want to be part of the project. Working with my colleagues, we identified leaders from various business and clinical areas to lead the working teams. I engaged our performance improvement and communications personnel to develop a mission, strategy, and a communication plan. We held a contest to brand the project; thus, CHOPtimize was born! In the early years, I provided guidance and direction to the teams, and I was their biggest cheerleader. Today, our CHOPtimize project has transitioned to an operational program. I am proud of the success of CHOPtimize. The level of engagement from leaders and frontline team members across the CHOP enterprise has been amazing. Today, CHOPtimize lives on and continues to be facilitated by Supply Chain with clinical and business leaders.

Your clinical staff will be able to suggest many supplies that are wasted, from extra linens in rooms that need to be laundered to supplies that often are tossed due to amounts or use issues. At our pediatric hospital, the IV start kit included an adult tourniquet that was often thrown away because a pediatric size was needed. As you take on this challenge, you will find lots of opportunities to ask your staff for ideas, such as:

- The cost of central line dressing care kits. (Do you use everything in the kit?)

- Office equipment, such as toner, paper, pens, and staplers. Consider reducing the number of printers by centralizing printing to control printer devices and ultimately toner costs.

- Medical equipment purchase and rental agreements for pumps and related supplies.

The nonlabor expense at CHOP is typically approximately 25% of the total operating budget and expected to be similar for a hospital or system. If you can reduce those expenses, it can go a long way to increasing the profit of your organization.

You cannot approach this effort with the goal of simply reducing expenses. Care for your patients and families should still—and always—be your primary goal. Encourage your staff to be innovative, and find solutions for complicated health problems. For example, our journey to control the cost of pulse oximetry began with a commitment to have accurate results for each patient. We learned to have different products for different patient needs and length of usage. We even introduced a more expensive, longer-lasting product for certain patients. We could demonstrate that giving the patient the right product results in savings. Sharing these examples with staff demonstrates our unwavering commitment to quality.

From the very beginning, you need to communicate the message that you won't be sacrificing quality of care or staff in the effort to reduce cost. Otherwise, you will not get staff on board with this process—a critical element to your success. The upcoming section, "Branding," covers how to create positive branding, and Chapter 5 offers advice on how to convince your staff that the goal is cost-efficiency, not simply reduction.

 NOTE

> Creating a culture of accountability is critical to the success of any healthcare organization. This requires a strong understanding of the complexities of healthcare, a balance of the many complicated factors that affect the quality of care, and a commitment from each member of the healthcare team to seek opportunities to drive improvement. Developing a program to foster active involvement of frontline staff in the judicious use of resources is one example of how a culture of accountability can be achieved.

An effort such as this one is ongoing, not short term. It can take a year or more from the time the operating plan starts with support services assigned throughout the year. Plan early.

The steps we followed, as shown in Figure 2.1, are:

1. Define the path
2. Develop the action plan
3. Align resources
4. Communicate
5. Celebrate success

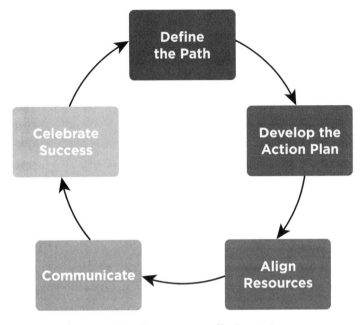

FIGURE 2.1 The steps to an effective strategy.

DEFINING THE PATH

Your path starts off with some paperwork, just like any project. Creating a mission statement, vision statement, goals, and branding sets the tone for the real work to come.

This is the first step needed to create a successful strategy. Exactly what will success look like? Think of it as the destination on a map that you can share with others to create a clear focus on the end destination. It's tempting to jump into action because there are many known ideas that will be part of your work. Stop yourself from jumping past this step because it will be needed as your true north star that will guide you and your team over time.

Vision, Mission, and Goals

Sure, your overall objective is to reduce expenses, but what else do you want to communicate about your effort? To make it clear from the start—with clinicians and business-people alike—it helps to develop a vision, mission, and goal statement pertaining to your savings efforts. These are the vision, mission, and goal statements we created:

> **Vision:** Think of your vision statement as what sets your long-term aspirations. It should focus on the future and be inspirational. We defined ours as:
>
> *To be the most trusted, reliable, and recognized Value Analysis Program that transcends traditional approaches in its relentless pursuit of safety and outcomes at an appropriate cost.*
>
> **Mission:** This is how you will achieve your vision. It is about what you need to do here and now to get there. We created ours to encapsulate two parts:
>
> *Together, we deliver value (world-class safety and outcomes at an appropriate cost) to patients and families through:*
>
> > • *Discovering and implementing new products and services safely and efficiently.*

- *Improving processes around nonlabor-related products and services.*

Goals: Define what success will look like to your organization and to your customers.

The goals/measures of success include:

- **Safety:** Product trials and implementations along with operational process improvements are completed with no safety events.

- **Value:** Both patients/families and clinicians will agree with the statement "CHOPtimize delivers value."

- **Financial:** Dollars saved will achieve the annual set budget targets and meet the overall target for nonlabor expense as a percent of net patient revenue.

- **Continuous improvement:** End users will be in agreement with the statement "The new product introduction process is effective," and the end user will engage in sharing ideas and join efforts to support continual improvement in clinical operations.

- **Culture:** Financial stewardship will be a key organizational pillar, with all staff engaging continually in the work.

Perhaps it would have been easier to simply say our objective was to reduce expenses. But we had higher aspirations; we wanted to shift the culture. We knew that we did not want to be a low-cost provider; we wanted to be the best provider for the kids and families. We purposefully crafted our objective and efforts around keeping and even increasing the value we brought to our patients.

By focusing on the value of your care and services, you engage with clinical teams in a different way. The discussion isn't simply about expenses—it can center on the quality of the goods and services compared to the cost of the goods and services.

Remember to keep your vision, mission, and goals visible and in conversation. This is something that you must demand and even add to your agenda items, or you can find yourself moving off course. This process also enables all the work teams to keep the same focus and maintain a shared message for consistency across the organization.

Branding

We wanted everyone to be talking about our program. We wanted to create a lot of energy and excitement around it, so we asked for help with the branding:

- Get the right people involved, from diverse areas of the hospital.

- Utilize a facilitator to spark conversation and capture all thoughts.

- Show examples of other known branding successes in all industries.

- Come back together in a second session with all the ideas and see what resonates.

To create the brand name, we ran a contest asking the team members for suggestions. We narrowed the recommendations down to three. We wanted a name that would resonate and be memorable. We spent time with our communications and marketing departments discussing each of the three options. We developed a few graphics and logos. Our final decision was based on the fact that CHOPtimize didn't have a negative connotation, it aligned with our values, and it was catchy and, yes, corny. It even became a verb. ("We CHOPtimized the copiers in our department.")

We had a lot of fun with the name; it was in everyone's conversation. On April Fools Day, we sent an email that stated that Webster's had accepted CHOPtimize as a new word in the dictionary...April Fools! Our communication plan had an event each month to keep CHOPtimize on people's minds. We tried to make each event, email, or story as memorable as possible, always acknowledging the work the teams had accomplished.

BRANDING WITH HUMOR

The typical didactic PowerPoint presentation is boring, and we wanted to instill tons of energy into this work to get people excited about saving nonlabor expenses—cost savings is not a really exciting topic for most. We wanted people to emotionally connect to our mission and make a lasting impression. We had to get creative. We had to tell a story. We needed to take a crack at starting a culture change.

We asked our Chief Financial Officer, Tom Todorow, to join us on stage and sit in a chair at the front of the stage. We provided him with a comfy pillow with images of $100 bills all over it. We shared with the audience that we borrowed it from his office, which created some laughter. It broke the ice.

We then told a story about how much each pulse ox probe costs and how often they are used intermittently and discarded after a single patient use. To demonstrate the pulse ox product, we attached Tom's finger to a pulse ox probe and a cardio respiratory monitor. We projected the pulse ox continual reading on the big screen for the audience to see his pulse and pulse ox reading. What the audience and Tom did not know was we had our simulation team behind the stage controlling the numbers displayed, so they were not Tom's actual numbers. At first, we showed a normal heart rate and oxygen level and commented how great of shape he was in. As the demonstration continued, we shared how we had opportunities to use a reusable pulse ox clip in some areas of the hospital, and we shared the cost savings between using a clip many times versus purchasing individual probes and putting them in the trash after each patient use. When we showed how much we could save, the simulation team dialed up his pulse, from 70 to 100 beats per minute. We commented that he clearly liked cost savings! Immediately people were laughing. We had one of our clinical nurse specialists come on stage and give him a water bottle and ask him if he was OK. Tom was laughing too, luckily. The simulation team slowly dialed back his heart rate numbers to normal, and we continued.

Our next point about the pulse ox probes was that they are recyclable. We shared the sheer volume of probes used each year and the dollar amount that could potentially be saved if we recycled the used probes with the manufacturer. Again, the simulation team dialed up Tom's pulse, but this time to higher levels of 120 beats per minute. This level caused the heart rate monitor to alarm, and laughter broke out across the room. This time, our CEO, Madeline Bell, commented how she never knew how excited Tom actually got about saving money, continuing that he always appeared calm on the outside. He just kept laughing.

At this point we did introduce the simulation team and their role in making these rapid heart rates happen. We assured all that Tom's heartbeat was actually fine. Most importantly, the message of taking risks, bringing humor, and engaging others became an underpinning of CHOPtimize.

DEVELOPING AN ACTION PLAN

An *action plan* is a written document that details definitive activities that must be performed well for you to meet your goals. It is best to create specific steps or needs so the plan is understood and void of confusion. Just like any long-term project, a cost-saving plan that will take years needs to be structured with a multidisciplinary approach. In any system—whether large or small—all disciplines need to be represented to generate a solid action plan that is applicable to all and doesn't require ongoing rework later.

Be sure to include high-level tasks, timelines, milestones, and resources in your action plan. Think about tools you'll need, such as tracking tools and a page on your intranet, a communication plan, and methods to keep the energy on the teams. Take a few months before the project kickoff to finish your action plan.

This step requires facilitated sessions with your leading sponsors to create a clear, concise, comprehensive plan. Including process improvement experts at this stage is critical for long-term support and team management. Open discussions and brainstorming activities will allow you to put everything on paper and then work through that information over multiple weekly sessions to keep momentum and energy around this activity. Don't get caught up in the details at this level. Focus on the major steps that must be taken, in which order, who is accountable, the timeline for each step, resources required, and how you will measure success. Putting the action plan into a schedule that can be easily accessed and reviewed often is critical to its acceptance and use.

Finally, keep revising your action plan until you have a finished version. Be sure to keep your group sessions close together to continue to advance your progress, and remember to return to your mission, vision, and goals to make sure you are including everything necessary to be successful.

ALIGNING RESOURCES

Traditionally, the cost of care is discussed at the executive level and in finance meetings, but not with clinicians, particularly with physicians and nurses. In any healthcare setting, clinicians are at the center of the care for patients. Physicians determine the tests to be run, the treatment plans to follow, and ultimately the discharge plan for patients. Nurses are at the bedside 24 hours per day with the patient, carrying out the full care plan.

Gaining the engagement of this staff is crucial to your success. As you start to identify resources for the program, think about the physician and nursing leaders who can serve as champions and influence their peers. These champions arise from your early adopters, who are inspired by the vision and take on a leading role to work actively with the team and be vocal about their excitement for the strategy. Not all adopters are good champions, though. Find those who want to make a difference and are hungry to show their value to the organization through such work.

On the flip side, consider the naysayers or resisters, too. Who do you think are the obstructionists? Who would be the devil's advocate? Put together strategies for working with those who were not immediately on board with your vision. It is often better to include them in your work teams to avoid future delay or negative impact after much work has been done. Listen to this group of individuals closely; their negativity may obscure a great point you should hear.

Another opportunity is to ask a vocal naysayer to work on an area of improvement or change that doesn't affect her specific area of work or concern, allowing her to see that this is a large organizational movement and not directed at just one area. In a large health system like ours, silos are often created, and individuals work hard to protect their area from outside critiques. Having a different set of eyes look at areas that they are not familiar with, such as a nonclinician observing a clinical area, is a great way to create areas of discussion and opportunity without intimidation.

The approach that we took was to have several multidisciplinary teams, all led by clinicians or business leaders, not by the Supply Chain department. *Multidisciplinary* can be best defined as staff that represent all clinical and nonclinical areas of an organization. Disciplines in healthcare are often used for only clinical or licensed staff, but we looked at all departments and staff across our system. The clinicians and business leaders consume the supplies and services; therefore, they are the best people to lead the initiative.

When your finance/consultant team hands you your organizational spend analysis, it will be clear where the high-dollar spend is occurring and on what items the spend is focused. This is your target area, which provides for the best and often easiest area of improvement. Our initial analysis identified the high-cost departments and categories as orthopedics, peri-op, and the emergency department, to name a few. Ask for dynamic, energetic leaders from these areas to take part.

Keep these points in mind:

- Choose natural leaders who can motivate others and push for innovative thinking and solutions, as well as sustain resilience throughout the initial phases of the program. The offer should feel like an honor to be requested to lead such a large organizational movement. We sent formal emails of request from the committee that added a more official component to the work.

- These leaders will need to assume additional responsibilities while continuing their regular work. It is imperative to confirm that individuals have the bandwidth to give the required time that has been clearly determined upfront and the enthusiasm to use their time on this team. Also, we required approval and agreement by the leader's manager.

- Compose small teams to brainstorm ideas. These teams should have a variety of staff to get different viewpoints. This selection was a critical part of the work. With the right people involved, not only could change be determined in the workgroup sessions, but the program could gain wide acceptance and involvement across the organization. Mixing clinical staff from all areas—pharmacy, nursing, respiratory, nutrition, with nonclinical staff from environmental safety, infection control, finance, and patient access—you create a dynamic in the room that invokes a questioning attitude. CHOP teams were kept to 12 to 15 members. We discuss brainstorming more in depth in the "Translating Organizational Vision to Work Team Efforts" section.

Remember to involve the Supply Chain department. They have valuable data that can provide direction to identify opportunities. Engage them as partners to help with supplier discussions, research for supply alternatives, and contracting experts.

COMMUNICATING

You need to get the word out—it is vital to get all employees working toward cost savings. When we developed the communication strategy, we used existing venues to target a broad audience.

Some ideas to try:

- **Hospital newsletter:** Use an existing newsletter to introduce your program, solicit ideas, and celebrate successes.

- **Leadership retreats and briefings:** These are the absolute best opportunities for your program to be advanced. A leadership audience supporting the same organizational goals and being asked to take these discussions and expectations back to their individual departments is a key area of impact.

- **Department meetings:** Spread the word at a more detailed level by attending department meetings across the organization and sharing ideas from other areas and possibly suggestions for them based on some proactive data review. Ask department leaders to establish a plan and goal for their specific department.

- **Events in your lobbies and atriums:** Add fun and excitement to your messaging by hosting tables with information and offering easy access to provide ideas, games, and giveaways.

- **System-wide emails:** Use your current communication pathways to continually share the work and stimulate employee engagement, awareness, and new ideas. Figure 2.2 shows a sample email.

Use the opportunities you have to start your program with high energy and enthusiasm, but remember to use these same avenues to sustain that enthusiasm and momentum throughout the entire program.

It was amazing to see the response we received about CHOPtimize. We received many emails with ideas. People started to use CHOPtimize as a verb. We also shared our program, vision, and branding with vendors during our usual business work. The CHOPtimize name became part of their language with us, and they quickly added opportunities to support our program through vendor initiatives and savings programs they could provide or had completed with other organizations. Spreading the word is essential to the success of the initiative.

To: All CHOP Employees
From: Joni Rittler, Vice President Supply Chain Management
Re: Paper Products (i.e., printer and copier paper) Ordering
         Process via Office Supply Store
Date: March 11, 2014

In a continued effort to identify additional ways to reduce expenses, we've begun to CHOPtimize our office supplies purchasing process. Following a recent review of our Office Supply Store orders, it was determined that we have substantial savings opportunities. The strategies to achieve these savings include:

- Reducing prices for current products
- Identifying best value items and utilizing automatic substitutions
- Enhancing departmental ordering using a customized CHOP shopping list

Paper products are our current focus for achieving best value for commonly used products. **By implementing brand standardization** (product from 14+ paper manufacturers is currently utilized with prices varying by up to 50%) **and auto substitution, the estimated annual savings for paper products used by CHOP is greater than $88,000.** Assessment of general office supplies and desktop printer toner will follow.

FIGURE 2.2   Use emails as a communication tool in your strategy.

After several months of detailed planning, assessing opportunities, and developing teams, it was now time to get to work. CHOPtimize was highly visible across the enterprise, and people were excited to be part of the effort.

 NOTE

> If you are an executive, be sure to give all the teams space and support while they get the work done.

The teams fed off of each other's level of enthusiasm. There was a light competitiveness that fueled the energy across the teams. For example, when linen utilization was being discussed as a large opportunity for savings, the different work teams provided their commentary on the reason they should include linens in their numbers. We all understood that overall savings was the goal, but we liked teasing each other over our savings numbers.

CELEBRATING SUCCESS

Give teams opportunities to see an early impact for their efforts. It will give them motivation to continue. It may also win over the resisters.

Try these methods to acknowledge the efforts and success of the teams:

* Have executives (such as CEO, COO, CNO, and Supply Chain Executive) visit and provide guidance and messages of support.

- Share teams' success stories at leadership briefings, in front of hundreds of leaders.

- Publish success stories in a weekly newsletter.

Over the course of the first year, we achieved more than $18 million in expense reductions, exceeding our goal of $15 million. We had an additional metric that we used to substantiate our efforts. We tracked nonlabor as a percent of net revenue. Prior to CHOPtimize, we had tracked around 26%; today we are at 24.5%.

BUILDING TEAM STRUCTURES

Building high-performing work teams is a critical step in the improvement work. After you have solidified the enterprise plan, it is time to move that plan into action. To do that you must first build your committee and team structure. In the earlier section "Aligning Resources," we talked about what kinds of people to fill your teams with; here, we talk about what kinds of teams you should have.

These teams work in parallel to each other and sometimes find opportunities to cross over or expand their savings project into another team. It is important for the leaders of these teams to create a supportive peer relationship to understand each other's projects and keep the team scopes clear. We also found that there were similar topics that affected all the work teams where this synergy was very helpful. These were often around topics of gaining access to a certain clinical division for discussion about product utilization, negative connotations regarding the CHOPtimize program as strictly a money-saving initiative, and even better ways to analyze the data to find areas for improvement.

Work Team Governance Structure: The Big Picture

You want to create a governance structure for your work teams based on how your organization divides opportunity categories. For example, an opportunity category is how you bucket your purchasing and spending. This structure is different for all organizations, but some basic work teams are Supply Utilization and Purchasing, Capital Expenses, and Purchased Services.

As you define each team, remember:

* Make your scope of exclusions clear, and adjust them as needed to not prematurely eliminate an opportunity. For example, including or excluding labor expenses would be a clear line that you would want to determine quickly.

* Think broadly and in all areas, clinical and non-clinical.

* Don't let your scope stifle unique ideas.

Team Leaders: Seek, Recruit, and Engage

It is important to look across your organization for team leaders who may not be the obvious choice at first glance. Perhaps this person is not a known leader to many, but someone who is closer to direct patient care and operational workflow, who has shown potential in some venue at your organization. Look closely at your newly appointed managers or directors, and you may be pleasantly surprised to find highly motivated and skilled leaders who are thirsty to carry an organizational initiative forward.

The steering committee spent time upfront having leadership discussions at the executive level to find the best candidates. They also had to gain commitment from the manager of those individuals before extending the request to ensure an adequate time commitment.

When choosing team leaders, look for:

- Strong individuals who bring different perspectives and insight to this work

- People with hands-on experience or organizational capabilities

- People with connections to help facilitate the ongoing work ahead

- People who can see the greater vision of work—one that is not solely a way to save money, but to lead a culture shift

- People with innovative ideas, even if not a content expert or clinician, who can broaden your scope of influence

- People who have displayed their ability to motivate a team

Team Members: The Backbone

After your team leads are in place, it is time to determine the committee members and structure.

Ask your team leaders who they would like to have on their teams. It establishes a strong collegial working relationship from the start. But remember that teams need to be inclusive across the organization.

Look for team members who are:

- Strong performers from many different areas

- People who understand detailed operations

- People who have nonbiased opinions and the ability to observe and ask questions that others may overlook. A new set of eyes looking at processes and analyzing data generates questions and discussions that may not have occurred with content experts.

Other very important members of this team include a member from your Supply Chain department who has immediate access to data and utilization information and a project manager who will support the administrative as well as the critically needed facilitative functions of a successful team. You need to have an established note taker to provide timely minutes, or you will find yourself starting at the very beginning at every meeting. We started by trying to have everyone take turns at recording and sending the minutes, but that failed very quickly. A single person, with a standard structure and clear follow-up actionable items and timelines, is integral to the team's movement. Ensure you have a process improvement expert fully involved with the team and guiding the improvement strategy along the way. This same person can be shared among multiple work teams. Structured improvement methodology ensures a comprehensive, data-driven approach to this work that can be replicated for each savings opportunity.

Members needed on the team include but are not restricted to:

- Nursing
- Supply chain
- Physicians
- Contracting
- Finance
- Infection control
- Process improvement
- Information technology
- Data sources: internal and external

To invite your chosen team members to be an official part of the team, create an official letter that explains the project work, how it is mission critical, and how it connects the enterprise plan to the well-being of your organization. Outline the goal of quality improvement, the elimination of waste, and the chance to affect ideas and actionable change.

Address the letter to the specific employee, and copy the employee's direct manager. Ask for the manager's support in allowing the employee to gain this experience and secure the time needed for this commitment. The employee has to accept and work within the roles and responsibilities that were established—most importantly the amount of time required to participate. Time expectations may actually eliminate some initial candidates from your group because it is often the case that people are already being utilized across your organization, completing their specific job functions and participating on many other committees. So, the litmus test for participation should begin with the individual's ability to truly give the allotted amount of time.

Topical Working Groups: Adding Specialized Input

All the work cannot fall on the shoulders of the team leaders and team members alone. To extend your reach, ask team leaders to create functional/topical working groups to gain insight and support for their specific project assignments. Follow the path of your work along the selection of a product, its procurement, and its use. Based on the actual project work, one or two additional colleagues could suffice for each working group.

For example, we created projects that focused on tracheostomy tubes, in which we pulled in a respiratory therapist to help understand the issues. Pharmacy leaders also spent time on a functional team evaluating and standardizing chemotherapy glove processes and brands.

Other, larger initiatives with greater impact may require more. When a functional group develops into a larger initiative, consider adding a project manager, Supply Chain member, or data analyst support to their work team.

Working Together as a Team

Your teams should meet on a regular basis—such as every other week—in the first six months to provide updates. These meetings can also serve as a time to educate team members on how to turn their project into a project plan, create a working group, navigate systems, and establish timelines.

Each team member can provide a verbal and written update to the group, discuss potential obstacles, and ask for help where needed. Spend time looking at your data analysis and determine the next item of focus and who could begin this work. We discuss many ideas in the later section "Translating Organizational Vision to Work Team Efforts."

Be sure to reassess and adjust your team over this extended project. Some team leads or members may get burnout or have less allotted time to give to the initiative. Show that it is OK to revitalize the group by transitioning in new members and allowing others to be thanked for their time and transitioned off. Ask them to continue to be positive vocal leaders from the front lines who support the change and educate their department community.

Hopefully you've chosen well and have the opportunity to grow some initial resisters on the team into your best leaders. If not, it may be difficult, but will be necessary, to ask them to step aside from their role by working directly with them and their manager to find a replacement member from their area or state that you are looking to expand into another area of focus at this time. These decisions are never easy but are vital to continue the movement of the projects and overall success.

CHANGING THE CULTURE

A big part of this challenge is undertaking a culture change. Begin with a clear vision, and set the expectations and goals. Then you must find your catalysts to promote the culture change. Look for those engaged leaders—the innovators and influencers—who can inspire the many followers needed to make a culture change. This critical step is all about identifying leaders who embrace the vision and are nimble at change:

- Recruit individuals who instill positive energy into the work and can build effective teams.
    - Arm them with data and give them resources to support the work.
    - Encourage them to create better processes and document them.
    - Help them educate staff and share results.
    - Create ways to recognize the contributors for their work.
- Have a steering committee; the leaders who are driving change can meet, share, and modify approaches to align with the vision.
- Be organizationally transparent, and create two-way communication avenues.
- Make presentations to staff to keep the messaging top of mind.
- Add electronic updates, from email to workstream blogs.
- Show organizational sensitivity to celebrate successes and learn from failures. In fact, embrace the lessons learned when outcomes are not achieved—it creates a safe space for others to try improvements.
- Message existing staff and new hires to ensure continuity in communication.

- Eventually embed the processes into operations once momentum is achieved. The quality improvement work and people you supported to change your culture now become your governance.

- Encourage continual organizational awareness about ongoing work. Make true commitments to monitor and support the sustain phase, because this is where the new culture lives.

TRANSLATING ORGANIZATIONAL VISION TO WORK TEAM EFFORTS

No matter how large or small your hospital is, the overall savings goal is most likely overwhelming to everyone. You need to take that large number and turn it into goals that your teams can accomplish. Ideas we used to break this down were categorizing high-volume products or processes that go across many departments, such as gloves or high-cost products that are used in specific areas, such as in surgery procedures. Another great focus is to review items that are ordered in many different sizes or package quantities and look to standardize by manufacturer or decrease the number of products in your inventory.

We came up with a few clear philosophies that became the CHOPtimize established plan. They are as follows:

- Identify, standardize, and analyze products and services

- Eliminate waste

- Uncover unnecessary costs

- Remove nonvalue-added features

Here are a few examples to start you on your way:

- Hold brainstorming sessions with preidentified groups to identify opportunities. These sessions can enable frontline workers to engage and share ideas.

- Assemble teams to work on common ideas. We had five teams, and each team had 12 to 15 members. Teams were intentionally kept small, and team members were expected to complete work between meetings. Each team had to vet the ideas presented to them from the brainstorming session; they were provided data to assist with the assessment. Also, the team members had to bring new ideas to keep a pipeline of projects. Overall, we collected more than 500 ideas on expense reduction opportunities. Chapter 5 outlines one such project.

- Perform walk-arounds in all areas of the organization. We observed differences in supply use among staff in the same departments as well as between departments. We also looked in the wastebaskets. Why were items thrown away that weren't even opened? What are we wasting, and how could we stop that waste? By simply looking around and asking questions, it was easy to quickly pick out issues that staff were dealing with on a daily basis. One clear example that was seen in almost all units across the organization was the fact that our glove box holders did not work properly; every time a glove was pulled out of the box, another glove would fall to the floor and needed to be discarded.

 NOTE

These expectations, however, cannot stand alone as the focused plan. They have to simultaneously maintain or improve efficiency, reliability, and quality. You do not want to turn your initiative into simply a money-saving campaign. At every point and every encounter, focus on how this work can improve your ability to provide services and improve the overall organization.

USING DATA TO DRIVE WORK TEAM FOCUS AND IMPACT

Your goal is to increase the value of your spend. To do that, you need to know where you are starting from. You need data. You can get this from your internal finance department or work with a consultant like we did to help break these raw data into useful information that can provide direction. What do your data show about your supply utilization? Look for identifiable items or categories in your purchasing data across the organization, rather than with an individual department.

Also, remember to check your data against external organizations. Choose like peer organizations that make comparisons easy; for us this was other children's hospitals. Be sure to look for opportunities of improvement, but also look at other nonlike organizations that can generate new ways of viewing this work. It helps to understand whether your culture and way of doing things could benefit from improvement that is happening at other organizations.

Aggregating this information is no easy feat. Having to create an internal system to capture and identify accurate information, pricing, and department-specific detail takes some time. But that time will serve you well because you can analyze the data in many different ways to support initiatives of change with clear information that can be shared with others. Look for:

- Obvious high-dollar, high-volume supplies, and establish leaders to take on specific projects around these items

- Places where you can easily trim expenses for quick wins that can help you add success stories to keep the engagement alive

- Short-, mid-, and long-term initiatives so you continue to see impact and results flow over the next year

- Pricing and product selection

- Standardization that can decrease waste and increase savings, both operationally and by item charge

 NOTE

Take all the ideas generated from the team and the employees during the walk-arounds, and merge them against the data to see whether the areas of noted concern really affect your supply information. Any matches can lead to eager team members who welcome a platform to move change forward.

3

ESTABLISHING THE "WHO": ENLISTING THE BEDSIDE NURSES

Megan Bernstein, BSN, RN, CPN, CCRN; Matthew Rutberg, Former Strategic Sourcing Manager, Supply Chain, and CHOPtimize Program Manager

WORDS & CONCEPTS TO LEARN

Fishbone diagram

Key driver diagram

Lean and Six Sigma methodologies

Nursing process

PDSA cycle

Process improvement

Project charter

Shared Governance

SMART goal

As touched on in Chapter 1, it is important to involve bedside nurses in a cost-saving initiative such as this. They are the frontline clinicians utilizing systems and supplies to provide high-quality care 24 hours a day. After your high-level team structure is created, it is time to involve bedside nurses to generate ideas for potential projects and empower them to take on the work.

Something that is immediately obvious whenever different types of people work together is that there is usually a clear difference in tone and verbiage between the groups. Because your cost-saving initiative involves executives who are responsible for healthcare business management and nurses who are hands on with patients, one of the first and biggest challenges you will face is how to create a common language between executive nurse leaders and clinical nurses.

Executives and clinical nurses can make a great team, and a culture of process improvement that delivers value to the bedside is possible. When both groups are open to learn from one another and can find common ground, creative and powerful approaches to problem-solving can lead to groundbreaking successes.

This chapter shows how to approach nurses through their existing organizations, how to involve them in meaningful and valuable ways, and how to bridge the disconnect in language. All of this goes a long way to engaging bedside nurses in the process.

TALES FROM THE FRONT LINE

My name is Megan Bernstein, and I have been a critical care nurse for over 11 years. I was looking to get more involved outside of patient care and wanted to contribute to positive changes in our hospital that could make a difference for our staff and patients. I was elected by my Shared Governance peers to be the Department Chair for the Supporting Practice and Management Committee within the Shared Governance program. It was a two-year reign with half of my time focusing on the work within Shared Governance and the other half of my time continuing my clinical practice as a bedside nurse in our Pediatric Intensive Care Unit. At the time, I had been a bedside nurse in my hospital for over five years, and although I was still incredibly invested in taking care of patients, I was ready for a new challenge. I had no idea what kind of doors this role would eventually open for me.

At the time that the CHOPtimize project was ready for bedside nursing involvement, my committee within the Nursing Shared Governance program, Supporting Practice and Management (SPM), was chosen as the right council for the job. As the Department Chair of the committee, I was able to meet with the Supply Utilization and Pricing leader first to discuss our initial steps in introducing the project to the nurses who sat on the committee. Truthfully, I was hesitant and apprehensive to attempt another cost-saving project after being involved in some in the past that were unsuccessful. As I sat in my scrubs, I listened to her talking, feeling slightly intimidated by her professional pantsuit. I was pleased to find that she was enthusiastic, approachable, and very easy to talk to. Within an hour of discussing the project with her, I was fully engaged. I knew my group of nurses were right for this work, and I knew that we could be successful.

INVOLVING AN ESTABLISHED NURSING COMMITTEE

Approach nurses through their existing programs, committees, and groups. CHOP has an established Nursing Shared Governance program, made up of nurses from all areas of the hospital to contribute informed decisions and improve and foster a collaborative work environment. Does your hospital have a similar group that can be an entryway to engaging nurses in the cost-saving efforts? Nurses are a vital component to reaching the goal, and they need to be part of the process as early as possible to help generate ideas for change. After all, they are the content experts. They should have input on the project charter, planning how the work will get done and setting timelines that will work for them.

An established program, committee, or group is the ideal way to engage the nurses. Find a group that:

- Has an established system to disperse information to other nurses.

- Best aligns areas of responsibility and streams of work.

- Ensures many or all areas of the hospital have involvement and nursing representation.

- Is made up of nurses who are already engaged in doing more to help their patients.

If your hospital has a Shared Governance program or similar group, look to see whether it will work for your program. If not, look around for another program or committee that aligns with it. Look for groups whose focus is related to workflows, financial stewardship, and operational systems.

In the past, CHOP had attempted several cost-saving projects, but they were unsuccessful. Nurses struggled to be engaged in the work.

CHOPtimize was different; it was set up to succeed with these elements:

- **A built-in structure:** Described in Chapter 2, have a clear action plan with goals and how to achieve them.

- **Executive level support:** Senior-level executives involved in the project should frequently make appearances at meetings to help answer questions and to hear about the progress of the work. Chapter 1 shares how to show executive support at the beginning of the project with elevator speeches.

- **Professional resources:** Assign process improvement advisors that are familiar with strategies and a methodology to collaborating and systematically approaching improvements and change. Utilize the various departments in your institution that have the right knowledge to help you, such as Supply Chain.

The executives know that involving bedside nursing in this project is important. Bedside nurses, after all, are the ones using the supplies every single day. They know where the processes are inefficient and where they are wasteful. Providing them the right resources and showing support is significant throughout the project.

EDUCATING NURSES ON HEALTHCARE FINANCE

A crucial step to introducing this project to nurses is to first help them understand why this work is important. Nurses have access to any supplies needed to care for patients. They are saving lives, after all! Whether an indwelling urinary catheter insertion kit is needed or a pack of gauze, nurses are attuned to using what's needed to provide quality patient care. Cost is normally not the main factor when it comes to using the supplies they need.

Most nurses are not taught about healthcare costs or healthcare economics in nursing school. Bedside nurses involved in committees or groups, such as Shared Governance, are usually nurses with three to five years of experience, with minimal exposure to this kind of knowledge.

Your first step is to give them some knowledge about the business side of the healthcare industry:

- Teach them about how the healthcare reimbursement through insurance and government programs works.

- Explain where your hospital stands in the healthcare industry. Hospitals having to lay off employees due to budget cuts can be used as examples of what can happen if expenses are not closely monitored and controlled.

- Emphasize that even though your hospital is financially secure, it is still at risk due to rising healthcare costs and changes to reimbursement processes.

- Keep language simple. Chapter 1 covers how to break down the big goal into smaller goals. It makes the work more relatable by comparing it to your home budget. Chapter 5 also has some tips on how not to overwhelm nurses with the big number.

Next, show them specifically the challenges involved in your hospital:

- Give them full access to the cost of your supplies and how much each specific unit spends on supplies. Nurses are always surprised at how much supplies cost.

- Ask them to start thinking about how many of the supplies are really necessary. How many pieces in a kit are thrown away? How many can be recycled or reused?

GETTING THE BEDSIDE NURSES INVOLVED

Now that your nursing committee or group understands what the mission and priorities are, it is time to take the project to the rest of the nurses. Nurses don't usually have much time away from the bedside to do extra work. You need a simple plan that everyone can initiate and that does not take away from their important work—their patients.

Find a way to keep up the momentum of the project by meeting with them frequently. Does the Shared Governance group or committee have a monthly meeting that you could attend? Ask for a small allotment of time at their meetings to help continue the work by answering questions and providing your support. The more time you spend with the nurses, the more engaged they will be in the work.

In the following sections, we give a couple of suggestions on how to generate ideas, so you can take the big concept—save money—and turn it into a full-blown project. Getting involved in a major hospital initiative can be daunting, especially if you've never done it before. Taking the time to walk them through step by step is part of giving them the support and resources they need.

NOTE

Transparency is important. Nurses should have the data to see where their money is spent. If you do not have real-time reports, ask for them from your Supply Chain department. They should provide details, including a list of the items being used, how much you are spending on the item per patient, and how much money the unit is spending overall for the item. If they do not know or understand what they are seeing, answer their questions. Offer educational sessions on these reports and how to break down and interpret the data.

Brainstorming Sessions

After the nurses are given the data, they now can start to brainstorm ideas about potential opportunities for cost savings. Make it fun. Use sticky notes. Encourage them that no idea is too small, whether it would save hundreds of dollars or thousands. You may only need one or two sessions to get the momentum going. It can be beneficial to meet in a big group so that ideas can build off each other. Hospital units can sometimes work in silos, so nurses having brainstorming sessions as a group may allow them to learn from each other and perhaps see things differently than before.

At CHOP, there was already a major project looking at pulse oximetry. So, this was used as an example. Every unit was clearly spending large amounts of money on pulse oximeters. Observe how, why, and when nurses are using a certain type of pulse oximeter. Ask yourselves and your nurses what works well with the current devices and what they think would make them better. Is there a different type of product that could be considered? Is there a way to recycle the probes so they could be repurposed and don't go in the trash?

These were exactly the types of questions that we encouraged the Shared Governance nurses to ask about their own supplies:

- It does not have to be the most expensive item or even the item most utilized on your unit. But where are you being wasteful?

- Where are you adjusting your workflow because of a supply versus the supply supporting your workflow?

Sit-Down Meetings

Some nurses will have ideas right away, and some will need help from you to find opportunities for potential projects. For those, schedule a sit-down to discuss their unit's workflow and supply usage. Ask questions, walk their halls with them, talk through their workflows, and assess their supply rooms. Chapter 5 goes more in-depth about how to conduct walk-throughs with the nursing staff.

And maybe it isn't a supply item you are wasting, but someone's time.

Generating Ideas

By now, you should have a number of ideas, and remember, no idea is too small. To help you generate thinking, here are some ideas we came up with for CHOPtimize:

- Linen utilization: Review when, where, and why linen is being used. Are there opportunities to use something instead of linen in certain situations? Are there opportunities to stock the rooms differently so that fewer unused linens are sent back for cleaning unnecessarily?

- Kits: Look at your pre-prepared kits. These are often put together to save nurses time and to avoid pulling individual supplies. Observe nurses using these kits. Talk to the nurses. Are there supplies in the kits that are frequently being discarded and, if so, why? Can you adjust the kits? Do you need the kit at all?

- Supply expense: Is a more expensive supply being used in scenarios where it is not necessary? Are surgical gloves being used when non-surgical sterile procedural gloves are a better fit for certain types of procedures?

- Supply waste: Are there scenarios where patients are moving from one location to another and brand new supplies are opened and subsequently discarded unnecessarily, anticipating their arrival? Could the process be modified to support doing the right thing and not being wasteful?

This is where a lot of nurses really start to get excited. They can see that a small change has the opportunity to make a difference.

After the nurses share their ideas, you can start to build upon them and move forward. Chapter 4 goes into detail on how to do this.

FINDING A COMMON LANGUAGE BETWEEN EXECUTIVE LEADERS AND CLINICAL NURSES

Because this was a high-level tactic with executive-level support, process improvement advisors offered help along the way. You will soon realize that executives, process improvement experts, and nurses do not speak the same language.

In fact, realizing this disconnect is a turning point. If the organization-wide project has a chance of succeeding, everyone needs to speak the same language. After you overcome the language barrier, you can then begin working as a team.

NOTE

> After you find a common language, do not expect that the rest of your cost-saving effort will go smoothly. There will be other obstacles to get through, but at least you know how to approach and talk to each other to resolve future problems.

For Nurses

We will not lie: You will hear a lot about charters, fishbone diagrams, SMART goals, key driver diagrams, PDSA cycles, and a lot of other things you will not understand and may not even care about. It can sound like a foreign language. However, improvement methodologies such as Lean and Six Sigma are quite similar to the nursing process, the process in which you care for your patients, as shown in Figure 3.1. These improvement processes are quite simply a strategic way of increasing efficiency and quality by eliminating waste and variability. It can be easy to get caught up in lingo and terms you may not have ever heard before.

As a quick reference, here are a few of the terms you may hear (some of them discussed further in Chapter 4):

- **Project charter:** The statement that defines the work you are trying to accomplish. This can include your goals, scope of work, and who will be participating in the work.

- **SMART** (*S*pecific, *M*easurable, *A*greed upon, *R*e-alistic, *T*ime-based) **goal:** An acronym for how to frame your goal statement and how you will achieve that goal.

- **PDSA cycle:** The method in which to test a change—**P**lan for testing the change, **D**o the change, **S**tudy how the change went, and **A**ct by either continuing with the change or modifying it.

- **Key driver diagram:** A visual tool for what will "drive" or contribute to the achievement of the project goal.

- **Fishbone diagram:** A diagram to help visualize the cause and effect of a problem.

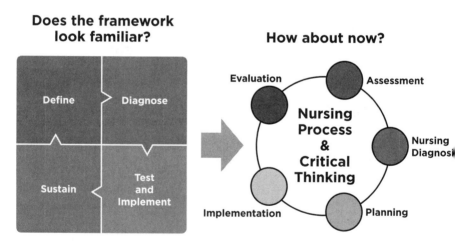

FIGURE 3.1 Process improvement methodologies are similar to the method nurses are already familiar with.

If you are a nurse working on this project, do not be afraid to ask questions. The executives and advisors that you are working with are not aware of what you don't know, and they will not judge you for clarifying your understanding of new information. They want you to succeed on this project, and starting off on the right foot by ensuring your full understanding of the work ahead is a step in the right direction.

For Process Improvement Experts

Nurses are the experts in their field. They know supplies and workflow because they live it every day. The success of this work depends on your ability to work together using the knowledge that both groups have. If you're an executive or improvement adviser, how do you know if you are drowning nurses in process improvement language they don't understand?

Some nurses may not feel comfortable saying so. What may come across as disengaged or uninterested may actually be a nurse who is not understanding the terminology. Be skeptical of nurses who don't ask any questions. They may not know the right questions to ask. In that case, ask them to repeat what their understanding is of the process step. Take the extra time to ensure they understand what is being asked of them.

Nurses do not lack process improvement experience and will not find the idea of process improvement challenging. Nurses actually are already process improvement experts; they simply use different words. You might think "nursing process" is slang, but it is the exact opposite: It's a formal methodology taught in nursing schools across the country and the world. The following table shows a few examples of the different language that process improvement experts and nurses use.

Process improvement speak	Nurse speak
Define	Assess
Tests of change	Interventions
Action plans	Care plans
Ad-hoc teams	Consults
Control the process	Evaluate and monitor

As you can see, the bridge to a common language isn't long, and the dream of building (or becoming) an army of process improvement experts at the bedside is not a daunting task. The Lean and Six Sigma methodologies used in the operations world are fairly similar to the nursing process. No one has to learn anything new; they—executives and frontline workers—just have to translate from one language to another.

Together, you can create and deliver a training curriculum that mirrors standard process improvement training. The differences include translation of concepts and terminology, with meaningful examples for nurses, and replacing widgets with medical supplies and bank loan applicants with patients and families. Moreover, you can use humor (self-deprecating at times) to further engage the group, bridge the gap between operations and nursing lingo, and reinforce main points.

 NOTE

Nurses are at a disadvantage by not being directly involved in healthcare finance from the very beginning. Bedside nurses not only have the clinical knowledge of supply utilization, but the dedication to their patients and motivation to improve the patient and family experience of healthcare. Not everyone you work with on a high-level project speaks the same language or has the same type of knowledge on the topic. But if you are open to new ideas, you can find your way.

ACCEPTING THE CHALLENGE

Accepting and embracing change is not something that should go underappreciated. For a bedside nurse, the financial world is new and unfamiliar—a major undertaking. This is an opportunity to learn something new, to grow your ability to be a well-rounded nurse, and to see that this ultimately is important for your patients as well. You might also find additional personal and secondary gains in this project—see Chapter 5 for some possibilities.

At the one-year mark from the start of this journey, CHOP had 28 active unit-based projects that totaled over $500,000 in savings and growing. This was a huge victory. It was thrilling to see that with the right support from peers and from high-level leaders and the right resources, nurses were trusted and empowered to lead the way and opened the door to a major hospital initiative.

 NOTE

> If you are frontline staff being tasked with this work, don't shy away from this opportunity. You can do—are already doing—this work every day. Simply put, no one knows more about supplies and supply utilization than you do. Take a chance on yourself and your ideas—you never know where they might take you. Share your success and failures no matter how big or small they are.

While this chapter highlights how to get bedside staff involved and the importance of utilizing similar language to communicate, Chapter 4 further breaks down the strategies and methodology used to move the work forward.

4

IMPROVEMENT METHODOLOGY: TRANSLATING THE "HOW"

Cheryl Gebeline-Myers, MS

WORDS &
CONCEPTS TO LEARN

Force multiplier

Gemba

*Model for
Improvement (MFI)*

Plan-Do-Study-Act (PDSA)

Process map

Project charter

*Total Employee
Involvement*

*Total Quality
Management (TQM)*

Practicing a disciplined approach to the science of improvement is important. However, it is easy for organizations to over-complicate the process. In theory, there is a "right" tool for every job; however, when working directly with busy bedside care providers, an approach that is focused on balancing structure and simplicity can prove more effective.

As you go along, you will learn a great deal about adapting the rigor of a chosen framework to leverage a high degree of frontline engagement and leadership of the change processes. This approach not only is effective in terms of nursing-led cost savings, but can also empower nurses in building their own capability to influence and lead structured improvement efforts throughout their careers.

TALES FROM THE FRONT LINE

My name is Cheryl Gebeline-Myers. I am a quality improvement professional with many years of experience in leading structured quality, patient safety, and process improvement initiatives. As the organization invested in the nursing-led cost-saving effort, I was brought in, along with a few additional colleagues, to implement a plan to engage bedside care providers in a structured approach to their efforts. This plan built on the crosswalk language outlined in Chapter 3. This approach had to be nimble and integrate just enough structure without overwhelming the nursing staff. We love all our tools and jargon in quality improvement, but in this case, it was a matter of ensuring we were leveraging just enough of these tools to drive a thoughtful, yet manageable, approach.

This reminded me of a time when I learned the valuable lesson around balancing form and function. I was a recent high school graduate and moving into my first apartment. I had a great foundation of life lessons and support from my parents to ensure I started off on the right foot. What I did not have was a tool belt—a literal tool belt, with hammers and screwdrivers. My mother was visiting, and I asked for her help in assembling my very first self-funded piece of furniture—a small pantry that came in what seemed to be a million pieces. My mother asked me for my "tools." The look on my face in response to this question led her to quickly think of Plan B. She is a nurse, and as any great nursing professional, she is quite "flexdaptable" when it comes to problem-solving in the moment. She asked for a high heel and a butter knife. Now these I had! We proceeded to put the pantry together with these "tools" quite effectively, and this pantry, now 20+ years and four moves later, is still standing. My father always says, "There is a right tool for every job," to which my mother responds, "But sometimes a high heel and a butter knife work just fine."

When you think of the science of improvement, the same lessons apply. You have fancy jargon, tools, and structured frameworks, but translating the "how" in a way that drives understanding and meaningful change at the bedside is the key to a successful endeavor.

THE SCIENCE OF IMPROVEMENT: A QUICK PRIMER

Improvement is indeed a science and discipline influenced by many great thought leaders over the years. W. Edwards Deming, known as the father of the Quality Evolution, had many notable contributions to the science of Total Quality Management (TQM). *Total Quality Management* is best described as a management philosophy used in customer-oriented organizations that relies on all employees having a stated focus on continuous improvement (American Society for Quality, n.d.). It is not a program or "thing" you do. Rather, it is an investment in a cultural transformation—one that values customers and employees, appreciates the role of systems and processes, and supports a model for continuous improvement every day.

The framework we used in the nursing-led cost-saving work fundamentally has its roots in TQM, coupled with the more practical, healthcare-focused Institute for Healthcare Improvement–adopted Model for Improvement (MFI). This framework outlines a cyclical improvement approach called Plan-Do-Study-Act (PDSA). The *PDSA approach* walks teams through structure planning, performing, and evaluating interventions within a given improvement project (Langley, Moen, Nolan, Nolan, Norman, & Provost, 2009). See the "Test and Implement: The Fun (Sometimes Really Hard) Stuff" section, later in this chapter, for more information.

To set the framework for success, TQM emphasizes several key elements that are instrumental to nursing-led cost-saving efforts at any organization.

There can be a lot of unfamiliar terminology as you undertake this important work. If you find yourself lost—whether you are an executive or a nurse—because you are confused by the language involved, turn to Chapter 3 to find out how to bridge the gap. You can find a common language!

Total Employee Involvement

Central to every single improvement effort are the employees—the very people who live and breathe the processes and systems (and their flaws) every day. An organization that does not consider Total Employee Involvement as a primary aim of its cost-saving efforts is one that will not maximize its cost-saving potential. This particular element of TQM is one of the most challenging. People inherently bring fear into any change process, whether consciously or subconsciously. This fear is particularly elevated in the context of targeted financial savings efforts. Employees hear cuts *not* savings and, understandably so, they worry.

In a healthcare setting, the perceived stakes and fears are exponentially higher. Your employees may have questions. "Does cutting costs lead to diminished quality of products, services, and care"? and "Will I have what I need to care for my patients?" These matters are paramount to frontline care providers. Their goal is to deliver the highest quality of care and experience for patients, and they may believe that cost savings means a compromise to that quality. How do you overcome that?

A strategy of Total Employee Involvement—one that involves all employees—will help win people over with this two-step process:

- **Reassure me:** Here you tackle the "fear" component. Through words and actions, assure your staff that you are leading with mission first. Focus on your branding of the work. Chapter 2 provides strategies on clarifying the mission and vision and successfully branding the work overall. How your employees feel and perceive the overarching effort is important to providing the assurance necessary for them to fully engage. It is important to emphasize that when employees participate in cost savings and waste reduction every day, they are in fact supporting a more sustainable, mission-centered outcome in the long term.

- **Tell me and show me:** Do not just tell your team that it is not about reducing the quality of care— show them it is not about reducing quality of care and then lead with this message in every presentation and discussion on the topic. For instance, you may encounter scenarios where a bedside nurse discovers that a more costly product is necessary for patient safety. Your receptivity to hearing this input and responding supportively certainly emphasizes your commitment to quality first. Tell them and show them at every opportunity, across all levels of the organization. Saturate this message in a very specific and purposeful way. It is indeed the most important message your staff needs to hear and see supported by actions.

Tackling these two needs first will set the stage for Total Employee Involvement in leading structured, cost-saving improvement efforts at the bedside.

TIP

If you are coming from a process improvement perspective, partnering with nurses to deliver value from the bedside can be one of the most exciting and rewarding experiences of your career. Challenge yourself to find creative and innovative ways to incorporate your operations and business expertise into their work, and empower them to make change rather than trying to lead it on your own. Help them to recognize and emotionally connect to the concept that reducing cost or financial stewardship does not equate to "cheap healthcare," but rather is a natural result of being patient-focused and making the most out of the organization's resources.

Process-Centered Focus

Another key element of TQM is an appreciation for the processes and systems that people experience every day. Improvement efforts routinely fail because they are tackled in a conference room by far-removed leaders versus at the point of the process with those directly involved. You would never sit in the boardroom and develop a plan of care for a patient you have never seen or one whose disease process you have not taken the time to understand. The same is true for when you undertake a cost-saving effort. Get input from the people who do the work day in and day out.

Take the time to understand the series of steps in everyday processes by directly observing frontline workers. Keep in mind that what people do and what people say they do is often very different. This is the power of direct observation. In cost-saving efforts at the bedside, it is important to avoid changing anything, such as a supply or piece of equipment, without first understanding the system and context in which it is used. You do this by watching its use in action, documenting the series of steps surrounding its use, and validating this with others. See Chapter 5 for a more direct description of this concept in action.

THE CHOP IMPROVEMENT FRAMEWORK: SIMPLE AND RELATABLE

One of the guiding principles for success in your cost-saving effort is to ensure the bedside team leverages a structured approach to their improvement work. While you should keep your approach simple and relatable, you should also set a standard and lay out expectations for the teams to follow.

The CHOP Improvement Framework is specific improvement methodology agnostic. This organizational improvement framework is grounded in concepts of TQM, MFI, Lean, and Six Sigma, and consists of four core phases: Define, Diagnose, Test and Implement, and Sustain (see Figure 3.1). You can easily incorporate this framework into your existing structure, as we describe in the next sections.

We committed to providing an adapted approach to leveraging the CHOP Improvement Framework—one that produced a balance between structure and feasibility for the nursing staff. We adapted our approach to training to align with already existing meetings. We selected a few key tools that we could teach in the moment, during already existing Shared Governance meetings. (Check out Chapter 3 for more information on Shared Governance.) We selected one phase per meeting, taught the basic tools, clarified expectations for completing this tool, and provided support and coaching as needed between meetings. This teach-and-apply method allowed the frontline Shared Governance representatives to tackle the structured improvement approach in a stepwise fashion.

 TIP

Acknowledge upfront the challenges that exist with busy clinical schedules. Listen to the needs of the frontline nurses, and be ready to adapt your approach. Ensure that it is not only relatable but also manageable. Consider when to step back from the rigor of your traditional methods.

Define: The Project Charter

The project charter is a core tenet to all improvement work. You can find a number of templates online for project charters, and no two are the same, but the principles are similar.

The charter is essentially the contract for the work. It includes the following elements:

- **The problem statement:** Describes the problem you are trying to solve or the opportunity you are trying to capitalize upon in an objective manner without commentary or opinion.

- **Scope:** What is and is not included in the work. This is often referred to as *in scope* and *out of scope*. Calling out these boundaries upfront is imperative to ensure the defined project and its scope remain intact. Veering outside of the defined scope can lead to scope creep, which can ultimately compromise the timelines and outcomes for the planned work.

- **Metrics:** How you intend to measure improvement. This is an important element for any improvement work effort. To answer this, ask yourself, "How will we know if the changes we make are resulting in improvement?" For nursing-led cost-saving work, you are best served to partner with your organizational resources to link cost or spend to your work and then track that over time. See an example of this in action in Chapter 5.

- There are typically three types of metrics in improvement work: process, outcome, and balancing metrics:

  - Process metrics are the measures to determine whether the processes you have put in place are being followed. Assume you put in a new process that requires support teams to round and refresh supplies in patient rooms every morning. Having a metric that captures whether this is being done every morning is a process metric. Process metrics are important to capture because as you often learn in improvement work, what you think is happening may not actually be happening.

- Outcome metrics are the "so what and who cares" metrics. These measures track the impact on system performance. At the end of the day, whether staff are performing the supply checks every day is not as important as understanding whether that change (or intervention) is affecting your unit's spend on supplies. Spend on supplies in this scenario is your outcome metric.

- The last type of measure are your balancing metrics. Balancing metrics look for potential unexpected impact as a result of your improvement work. For example, the time that the support staff spend on rounding may mean that other important work for which they are responsible is not getting done. Having a measure that focuses on potential other or downstream impact allows you to keep an eye on this.

- **Risks and dependencies:** The risks and dependencies you anticipate are important to acknowledge early in improvement work. A *risk* is a known factor that could get in the way of your improvement work. A common risk is competing priorities. It is important to call this out and discuss ways to mitigate this risk toward the beginning of the work. A *dependency* is more of a "what must go right" framing, or what other factors are in play that your work could be dependent on. For example, in nursing-led cost-saving work, being able to measure the spend for your project is important. Thus, having a system to track supply cost may be an overall dependency for your improvement work.

- **Other key factors:** The charter also captures other important details, such as people who need to be involved, timelines, and deliverables. The charter process also requires a review from others to gain support and sign-off for the scoped work. This sign-off is an important commitment for the work to be performed. The charter is typically drafted by the person or people more directly carrying out the work, but the charter discussions, review, and sign-off often involve relevant leadership whose guidance and buy-in are necessary to support and influence the work. Everyone must agree to the project charter terms in the beginning.

The project charter (see Figure 4.1 for an example) provides a continued framing and reference point. It is not a "once and done" document and often needs to be revisited as the improvement work evolves. The charter is more of a process than a document; the most important components are the discussions you have around the overall purpose of the work and the commitment necessary to support its success.

Diagnose: The Process Map

The next step is to create a *process map*, which is the process of breaking down all your activities to determine how they flow and, ultimately, how effective they are. Process maps make you scrutinize every element in your process, what's absolutely necessary, and where the waste or problems exist.

Process mapping can seem to be complicated and time-consuming to tackle, something a lot of people will not want to do—especially when they are trying to fit it in between caring for patients. But it doesn't need to be. Nor does it need specific shapes or symbols or to be created with fancy software. Scrap paper works just as well as PowerPoint.

What matters most is the fundamental understanding of the process that's being mapped. To show everyone that they too can process map, try the following points:

- **See it to believe (and understand) it:** In process improvement, this is called a gemba walk. *Gemba* is a Japanese term that means "the real place," or the place where the work is happening. Encourage people to directly observe work to map the process in its real state, not the perception of how the process works or should work.

Project Title				
Team				
Executive Sponsor(s)				
Sponsor(s)/ Team Leaders				
Improvement Advisor(s)				
Team Members				
Project Purpose				
PROBLEM STATEMENT What is the problem to be addressed?				
MISSION/STRATEGIC PLAN Why is this project important to the organization?				
METRIC(S) How will we know a change is an improvement?				
IN SCOPE Why is this project important to the organization?				
OUT OF SCOPE				
KEY DEPENDENCIES/RISK(S)				
Timelines				
MEETING FREQUENCY				
DECISION MAKERS Who needs to be at meetings				
Goals	**Define**	**Diagnose**	**Test & Implement**	**Sustain**
Completion Deadline:				
Signatures – Project Start				
Executive Sponsor			Date	
Sponsor(s)				
Improvement Advisor				

FIGURE 4.1   The project charter.

- **Tell me the "right" way:** While process mapping is one of the basic quality improvement tools, there is not really a "right" way to process map. When you talk to the frontline staff about process mapping, place emphasis on the "why" and do not worry too much about how it's done.

The efforts of the frontline nurses led to colorful and creative process maps; some used symbols and PowerPoint, and others simply created sketches on a sheet of paper. Regardless of the method, every map was effective in its intent to understand the process in its actual, versus perceived, state. Figure 4.2 shows a few of these process maps.

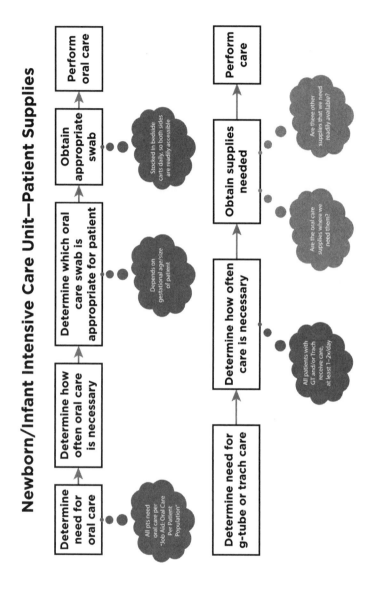

FIGURE 4.2 A few creative process maps.

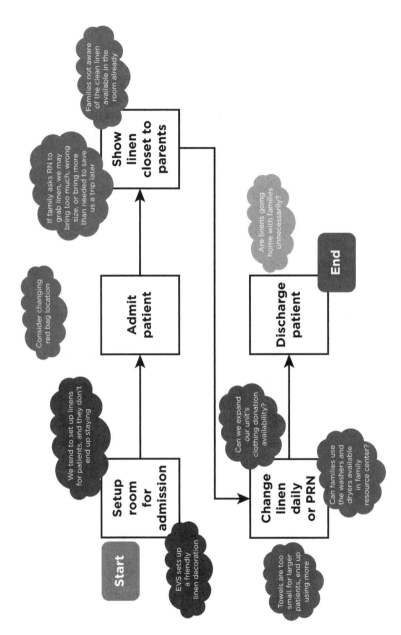

FIGURE 4.2 A few creative process maps. *(continued)*

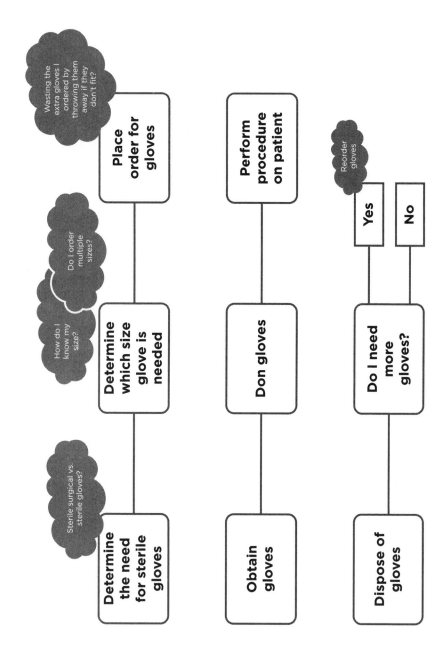

FIGURE 4.2 A few creative process maps. *(continued)*

96

Test and Implement: The Fun (Sometimes Really Hard) Stuff

Leveraging the project charter and process map, you can move on to the Test and Implement phase.

Encourage your members to "think big, test small." With this approach, they can come up with a big idea but test it in a small way to see whether it has the potential to work on a larger scale. Chapter 5 provides a great example of this in action. Doing so helps members not become quickly overwhelmed by trying to make too much change or tackle something too big early in the process. Focusing on a small pilot or test also helps you decide what the next steps to take are and gain traction on tackling bigger ideas. Testing small can be a difficult concept for teams to embrace, but it can decrease anxiety levels and increase confidence.

 NOTE

"Think big, test small" also allows small victories and chances for success early on in the process, which helps employees understand that this process works and encourages them to continue.

During the Test and Implement phase, the Plan-Do-Study-Act (PDSA) approach works well, which is one of the tools in the CHOP Improvement Framework. PDSA is a commonly used approach to improvement projects and one that easily translates to the bedside staff. Figure 4.3 shows an example. Follow these steps:

- **Measure-Intervene-Remeasure:** Use data to understand where you are in the current state (pre-intervention). Initiate your changes and remeasure to understand the impact of the change.

- **Adopt-Adapt-Abandon Change:** After reviewing the impact of your small test, you must decide how to proceed:

    - *Adopt:* For changes that had an impact, were received well by staff, and overall improved the quality and/or cost effectiveness of your work, continue on a larger scale.

    - *Adapt:* For changes that had some impact, but not entirely where you wanted it to be, tweak your test and rerun it.

    - *Abandon:* For interventions that had little to no impact or were particularly challenging to see working in the long run. Encourage teams to develop thoughtful tests but to not be afraid to fail. It is all part of the process. In improvement, you will want to "fail fast" so you can integrate lessons learned, restrategize, and approach the problem from a different angle.

The Test and Implement phase generates the most hands-on activity and provides a great opportunity to convince the resisters that the cost-saving effort is worthwhile. This phase is where your team leaders need to provide ongoing encouragement to the early adopters and coax along the doubters.

It is also important in this stage to prepare for resistance. A common issue in any change, resistance can derail progress if it is not handled properly. Some tips:

- Do not be discouraged by resistance.

- Seek first to understand. Speak directly with people about their concerns. You can often learn the most about issues that have the potential to impede success overall, and you can try to mitigate those potential failure points.

- Take the opportunity to pause and reflect on your approach.

- Leverage open-ended questions to learn what others think about your planned improvement approach.

You can also use this as an opportunity to engage those who are concerned overall. While not always the case, sometimes their concerns represent an interest in the success of the work, and capitalizing on their interest can be helpful.

Throughout the work, but most importantly in this Test and Implement phase, use resistance as an opportunity to be a positive role model for change. It might not just benefit the improvement work, but also your own professional development as well.

PDSA WORKSHEET

Project Name:	Date of Test:	Cycle: 1 of X
Overall team/project aim:		
What is the objective of the test?		

PLAN:
Briefly describe the test:

How will you know that the change is an improvement?

What driver does the change impact?

What do you predict will happen?

DATA—Describe the precise methods for collecting, validating, & analyzing data	Person Responsible	When	Where
Baseline Data:			
Test of Change Data:			

TASKS: List the tasks necessary to complete this test of change	Person Responsible	When	Where
1:			
2:			
3:			
4:			
5:			
6:			
7:			
8:			

Plan · Do · Study · Act

FIGURE 4.3 An example of a PDSA worksheet.

Sustain (and Spread!) Successful Change Efforts: Sharing Is Caring

The last phase is to sustain the effort—embed it in the everyday operations. That's easier said than done, of course.

Sustaining change efforts requires a thoughtful approach to integrating the new process into your day-to-day work. This may include any combination of policies, procedures, processes, or layout changes, hard-stops, education, and reinforcement. These new processes and changes should be easy for people to understand and follow in the future. The Sustain phase typically includes planning for continued measurement to ensure the new change or process remains "in control." That is, you are not showing a return to former practices, and you can sustain the improvements moving forward.

Chapter 5 includes a great example of integrating the improvement work into daily operations—essentially "how we do things here." In this example, following a small test and the decision to "adopt" the change into operations, modifications were made to every patient room on the unit to ensure the supplies were organized and available when needed. This is an example of changing the layout of the room to ensure sustainment of this new process in the future.

As your nursing-led cost-saving efforts evolve, you will likely encounter an important question. How can we share and spread best practices across units? The Nursing Shared Governance council at our hospital requested a tool for this.

Developed by improvement partners, this tool (see Figure 4.4) allows nurses to "tell the story" of the improvement— what worked, what did not work, what to keep an eye on, and how to measure. Sharing these across units can break down silos between units and create a force multiplier for your overall cost-saving work.

The nursing-led savings work presented a unique challenge to our improvement approach overall. As an effort led by Nursing Shared Governance, there was great interest in not only implementing change, but also spreading successful interventions. In an attempt to bridge connection between units and initiative, we focused on developing a flexible tool that allowed units to document their change efforts, people involved, issues encountered, keys to success, and overall impact of the change. These were then stored centrally for leaders and other Shared Governance representatives to access to identify potential opportunities to spread the change to their area as well. This created a *force multiplier* (something that increases the production or effectiveness of a process or team) and broke down silos between units.

SPM IMPROVEMENT SPREAD WORKSHEET

Initiative Proposed for Spread: _____

Successful Department: _____

Department Representative: _____

Implementation Period: _____

Area(s) Identified for Opportunity: _____

Approved by: _____

Background
- What is the improvement opportunity?
- What test of change are we trying to spread?

Evidence/Data
- What evidence or data shows the success of the project to spread? (Insert graph/chart if applicable)
- How will success be monitored? (Metrics)

Impact
- Why should this initiative be spread?
- What will be the impact to:
  - Your area?
  - Patients?
  - Workload?

Implementation Plan
- What people (internal/external) need to be involved?
- What is the time needed to implement?
- What will the method be for measuring impact?
- What are the steps needed to implement this change?

Challenges/Barriers
- What challenges and barriers do you anticipate in implementing the improvement? (e.g., time, resources, financial constraints, etc.)

FIGURE 4.4   Improvement spread worksheet.

Additional Comments:

Implementation Timeline (To be completed by department implementing improvement)

Phase	Start Date	Target Completion Date	Actual Completion Date
Define			
Diagnose			
Test & Implement			
Sustain			

NOTE: Please attach the final version of the Improvement Spread Summary with a PDSA Worksheet for the improvement being spread from the department that recommended the spread.

FIGURE 4.4 Improvement spread worksheet. *(continued)*

REFERENCES

American Society for Quality. (n.d.). What is Total Quality Management (TQM)? Retrieved from https://asq.org/quality-resources/total-quality-management

Langley, G. L., Moen, R., Nolan, K. M., Nolan, T. W., Norman, C. L., & Provost, L. P. (2009). *The improvement guide: A practical approach to enhancing organizational performance* (2nd ed.). San Francisco, CA: Jossey-Bass.

5

NURSING-LED SAVINGS IN ACTION: A BEDSIDE NURSE'S PERSPECTIVE AND STORY

Jessica Steck, BSN, RN, CPN

WORDS &
CONCEPTS TO LEARN

Cost per item

Fiscal year

Patient days

Spend and utilization charts

Unit spending trends

By now you have learned a great deal about the organizational approach to CHOPtimize work (see Chapter 2). Various high-level employees did a bulk of the prep work before bringing the project to Shared Governance and the other frontline nurses (see Chapter 3).

In this chapter, we explain how you can go from an idea (can we spend less on glucose testing strips?) to trial (will a dedicated storage bin help?) to execution (taking the storage bins unit-wide) successfully.

TALES FROM THE FRONT LINE

My name is Jess, and I have been a nurse since 2010. I have worked on the same floor at the same hospital since earning my nursing degree. At the start of the CHOPtimize project, I was exclusively a frontline nurse. I spent every day in direct patient care. My three 12-hour shifts were spent assessing patients, attending rounds, giving medications, changing dressings, checking blood sugars, placing nasogastric tubes, and more. Hospital expenses were at the very bottom of my priority list, and if I am being honest, they were not really on my list at all. Never once did I think how much gauze, gloves, or masks cost the hospital. I believed that kind of work was for executives and business people. I was far too busy with all the tasks that take up a nurse's day to think about how I could make an impact by saving a couple of dollars.

All of that changed when my journey through the CHOPtimize program began. I realized that the decisions that I made on a day-to-day basis do make a difference in the bottom line of the financial welfare of the hospital.

At the time I started with the CHOPtimize team, I was a brand-new unit member of the SPM Shared Governance council representing my 35-bed combined medical subspecialty unit with patients under Endocrinology, Liver

Transplant, Gastroenterology, and Metabolism services. When I attended my first CHOPtimize meeting, I was overwhelmed by the idea that I had anything to contribute. Turns out, I did. Even though this world of financial cost savings was new to me, I was struck by the enthusiasm the team brought to the idea of nurses leading cost-saving projects in all the individual units. It was this enthusiasm that helped me to become an early adopter.

If you told me back in 2010 when I graduated from nursing school that I would be writing a book on nursing-led financial stewardship, I think I would have suggested that you seek the help of a medical professional. All of that changed when the CHOPtimize team presented their work in a fun and light-hearted way at my very first Shared Governance meeting. I could have taken on this project, given it a halfhearted effort, and called it a day, but for some reason I took a chance on myself and believed I could do it with the support of my unit and peers. Whether you are part of the administration or part of the frontline staff, take a chance on yourself and believe that you and your organization can do this, too.

I, Jessica Steck, a bedside nurse from the suburbs of Philadelphia, have presented my story and the work of this team at national and international conferences, and now I am writing a book about it. PINCH ME! This project has brought me so much success and professional development over the last few years, and I will really be forever grateful for the opportunity to work on it. I'll never forget the day I booked my conference and airfare tickets to sunny Florida to present at a conference when I realized I had no business casual clothes. I wore scrubs on my work days and yoga pants on my days off. I stumbled through the mall going through department stores looking to trade in my clogs and scrubs for dress pants and flats for just a week. Those dress pants and blouses have been put to use many times since that day, and I am grateful for the help of the sales associate in the store for being patient with my complete lack of knowledge of dress pant styles.

STARTING THE WORK

It is easy to be handed a task and put it at the bottom of your to-do list, especially if it is not related to patient care. And looking at confusing financial charts and graphics that highlight your unit's spending history might lead you to put this work further down your to-do list. As a bedside provider, you might be thinking to yourself, "How can I make this work a priority while I have so many other competing tasks in the day?" Here are a few tips:

- **Partner with the leaders on each unit.** If this work is made a priority and is supported throughout the institution, you should be given time outside of patient care to support you in executing ideas into plans.

- **Use downtime.** As a nurse who has been at the bedside for eight years, I know downtime is very hard to come by. While you explore options for where or how you could save, use time with other staff members to brainstorm. Whether in the lunch room or at the nurses station, start discussing supplies and waste, and the ideas will start flowing.

- **Keep the idea of financial stewardship in your mind always.** Though you might not have the time in a specific moment to formulate a plan, keep track of ideas you have throughout the day. Note when and how you use products and any ways you think that could be improved.

- **Speak up!** Tell someone about those ideas you have. Tell your manager, a supervisor, or a nursing leader.

Now you have been given a bunch of data, and that can be overwhelming, but even if you are not financially inclined, that does not mean you are not up to the challenge. These lists might be long and confusing, so take it item by item. Look at how much an item costs *(cost per item)*, how long patients stay *(patient days)*, and unit spending trends or history *(how much your unit uses an item over time—per quarter or per year)*. When given access to data like this, look at it with your lens as a nurse. Look at these numbers the way you do vital signs or lab values. Do they make sense for your population? Are you surprised by anything? The nursing process and the process of improvement continue to align.

For example, glucose testing strips were at the top of the expense list for my unit. On the Endocrinology, Liver Transplant, Gastroenterology, and Metabolism services unit, many patients have their blood glucose levels checked anywhere from a few times a day to every 10 minutes when they are undergoing various diagnostic studies. These little tiny strips are used constantly. Was it surprising to see them on the top of the unit's spending list? No. Was it surprising to see how many were used in a three-month period of time? Absolutely.

This was one area that my unit identified as a potential supply that we could save some money on. With the CHOP Improvement Framework (which you can read about in Chapter

4), in less than a year, the Endocrinology, Liver Transplant, Gastroenterology, and Metabolism services unit cut the number of glucose testing strips used by 98%, leading to an annualized savings of over $35,000. By identifying areas of waste and storage issues, we were able to identify an opportunity for improvement.

Remember that most nurses don't have a financial background. If you need a frontline nurse to understand a financial term like utilization charts and unit spend trends, define them and explain the difference one or two things can do to affect the bottom line. I recall looking at the PDF I received at one of the initial meetings—20 or more pages of lines and numbers next to supply items. I was overwhelmed and had mounting questions:

- Why did this chart start in July?

  - The idea of a *fiscal year* (a designated 12-month period companies use for budgeting, forecasting, and reporting) was brand new to me. I highlight this very basic educational point to help bridge the gap between upper-level management and the frontline staff. Start with the basics.

- How can I digest all the information in the document, and where do I begin?

  - Thankfully, the leaders of this work anticipated these types of questions and feelings. A

large portion of our initial meeting was devot-
ed to just understanding the very basics of our
unit's data. If you are a frontline staff member,
attend these informational sessions. If you are
a leader, host them.

- Speak up!

  - I know I've said this before, but it is worth
    repeating. If you have a question, odds are you
    are not the only one who doesn't understand.
    One of the keys to the success of a large-scale
    project like this is open communication. The
    leaders may have no idea the data are confus-
    ing to staff if someone does not speak up.
    Reach out to the leaders of this work, nurs-
    ing or otherwise. Is there a person from the
    finance department on the team? Can they
    help to translate this financial jargon into ev-
    eryday language? Does the nursing leadership
    supporting this work have tips or a toolkit to
    help the bedside staff involved succeed?

The next section, "Avoiding Getting Lost in Translation as
a Nurse," goes into more detail about helping your frontline
nurses not be overwhelmed by the financial concepts.

AVOIDING GETTING LOST IN TRANSLATION AS A NURSE

So, how do you engage frontline staff in the process of ongoing financial stewardship when they may have never even heard the term "financial stewardship"? Using language that everyone—clinical and nonclinical staff—can understand and the correct messaging is how this work gets done.

Chapter 3 goes in-depth on this topic, but here are some key points to help make nurses more comfortable:

- Financial stewardship is a big term. Break this, and other business terms, down to a level that staff can understand. Know that the majority of your staff does not have a business background, but they do have the same goal you do every day—providing the best patient care they can. Therefore, teach financial stewardship as not just a line of numbers but a means to achieve high-quality patient care. Ultimately, then, everyone can become a steward of your mission.

- The goal is to cut "nonlabor expenses," which means not cutting staff. This message was the most important to me from the very beginning. The goal is to manage nonlabor expenses, such as eliminating supply waste and finding the right products for the right task. Cutting staff was *never* a priority.

- At the time of this project rollout, the local news talked about hospitals in our area having to cut their workforce. Nurses on the front lines of patient care know the importance of every single member of the healthcare team. More nurses and ancillary staff are usually needed, not fewer. Get the nurses thinking about how to save money, not their jobs.

- One person alone won't save a million dollars, but everyone together can. Imagine what could happen if every employee is able to save a few dollars a week. The cumulative cost savings could be huge. Whether you work at a small community hospital or a major academic medical center, the cost-saving potential can be significant.

- The goal is not to find the cheapest products. When the CHOPtimize program was launched, there was a misconception that it was only about cutting costs. The goal of the project was to decrease costs while increasing the value of patient care. If an expensive product fits your needs and helps prevent hospital-acquired infections or injuries, it is worth keeping. Those sorts of products are, in a sense, priceless.

- Ask your frontline staff; they are already doing the work. Get the nurses to think about the day-to-day actions they take. For example, the nurses at CHOP often threw away the gloves that came in a specific kit and used a second pair of sterile gloves that fit better. These gloves in the kit were "one size fits all," and almost no one likes how they fit. All the nurses knew this, but members of the Supply Chain who ordered these kits did not. Removing the gloves from the kit allowed staff to obtain the gloves that fit them best prior to the procedure and eliminated wasting the second pair of gloves. This was an easy way to make a big savings impact, but not one that executives would have realized if they had not asked the nurses.

- Ask nurses to think about their own household budgets. In your personal lives, you are all trying to save money. From cutting coupons, shopping at discount stores, to buying in bulk, you all make efforts to save a few dollars. The same thinking can translate to the hospital.

- Be aware of the naysayer. Staff had a lot of questions and thoughts when the CHOPtimize projects began. "They want me to save on a pair of sterile gloves, yet we are building a multimillion dollar building right across the street." Address the elephant in the room (or across the street), and educate the staff on the state of healthcare in the United States and in your local area.

- Be enthusiastic about this work. Hospital finances are boring. You can make them less boring and more approachable by bringing fun and humor to the presentations. CHOP had executives giving elevator speeches to the nurses—60 seconds to convince a group of nurses that they should care about the financial state of the hospital and healthcare. These types of executives are used to having the captivated ears of hundreds at town hall meetings, and here they had only one minute to tell the nurses why they should be invested in saving the hospital money.

WALKING THE WALK

We've all seen the cartoons depicting nurses with several sets of arms trying to balance all of their daily tasks. Ask the average staff nurse if there is enough time in the day to get all the tasks and documentation done, and the answer is almost always a resounding "NO!"

Show nurses how they can incorporate this additional work into the daily work they're already doing. In this way, you are not asking them to reinvent the wheel. The nurses are the absolute experts on the day-to-day utilization of patient care supplies. One approach is to follow a nurse gathering supplies for a procedure. Ask:

- Is there something about this kit that isn't helpful or isn't used?

- Is one type of supply used for one or more purposes?

- Is there a favorite or least favorite supply in the kit? If so, why?

- Is there a supply not in the kit that should be included?

The staff may feel skeptical about your interest in their day-to-day work. They might wonder why an executive or leader is following them around asking about supplies. Be open and honest with them from the very start. Tell the staff members you are not an expert in patient care supplies, and that, in fact, they are. Use open and honest communication. This is a great time to dispel any of those rumors mentioned earlier (e.g., you are not just looking for cheaper products). Hopefully, the staff will appreciate your general interest in their work and their process, and you will gain a lot of insight during this short time.

The most time-consuming and challenging work for the frontline staff leading these efforts comes after they have identified supplies that could be removed, improved, or updated. Like financial stewardship, the term *process improvement* is new to much of the frontline staff. You read in Chapter 3 about how the nursing process and process improvement framework are very similar. Continue to use this message to encourage staff along the way to create and execute ideas that could lead to meaningful changes.

CREATING A PROCESS MAP

After you have an idea or two where you can save some money on your unit, sit down with the other nurses on your unit to discuss how the item is used. Creating a process map helps you lay out how, why, and when an item is used and if or where there is waste involved.

In the early-morning hours of one of many night shifts, I sat down with co-workers and started to talk about how we use glucose test strips. At some point between feeding patients and doing assessments, I created a process map, or the walk-through of my product utilization, and discovered a ton of product waste, shown in Figure 5.1. To do this work did not require a lot of effort. I did not feel the pressure to complete a process map that was perfect or of the highest standards in process improvement. I knew that the leaders of the project just wanted my ideas and my suggested improvements. Whether I had the right colors, shapes, or arrows did not matter. See Chapter 4 for more information on process maps.

For the glucose test strips usage on my unit, a problem revolved around their availability at the bedside. A patient's blood glucose level needs to be checked at a moment's notice. We did not have a standard place for the testing supplies. When it was time for discharge, three or four half-filled vials of test strips would usually end up in the trash or

in the miscellaneous drawers at the nurses station (and ultimately in the trash). This was a huge waste of product.

Process Map: Glucose Test Strip Utilization

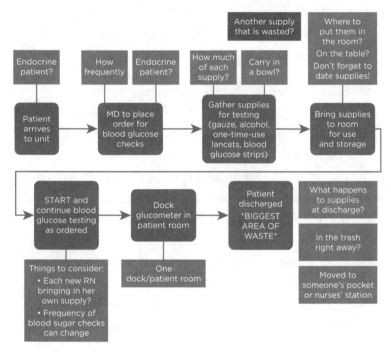

FIGURE 5.1   One process map.

FOLLOWING UP ON INSIGHTS

Next, think about how you can prevent waste or inefficiencies from happening. In the case of the glucose strips, why

not have a uniform place to store supplies? What if all the glucose testing strips are kept in a place that also holds all of the other needed supplies for checking blood glucose level (alcohol swabs, gauze, one-time-use lancets)? The solution was a storage bin—one that was wall-mountable (thus out of the reach of small curious children) and made of a hard plastic that could withstand cleaning—that could store all the glucose testing strips in one place.

HELPING YOUR STAFF TO NAVIGATE YOUR OWN HEALTHCARE SYSTEM

Navigating the healthcare system is difficult. You have an idea, and you are ready to execute it.

 NOTE

> Here is where you have to exercise patience. As a nurse, you are accustomed to seeing results right away. You have a diabetic patient with high blood sugar; you give her insulin, and you see improvement right away. When implementing wide-scale change, approvals cannot happen overnight. Don't abandon your work just because it is taking a while to get things moving, and don't be afraid to be persistent.

You'll need to meet with key stakeholders and gain their approval for your ideas. From facilities, infection prevention, regulatory readiness, and point-of-care lab, you'll be meeting with people, making connections, and sharing your ideas.

There are many people within the hospital setting you will need the support of for a project to be successful. A few key stakeholders and why you might need their support are:

- **Facilities:** If any equipment will be added or removed from the patient environment, you will need the help of the facilities department to make this happen.

- **Infection prevention:** It is always good to loop in the infection prevention team when it comes to adding something to the patient environment. Anything that stays in a patient room between patients will need to be able to withstand cleaning.

- **Environmental services/housekeeping:** Again, if an item is being added to the patient environment, it will need to be cleaned between patients. It is important to make your environmental or housekeeping department aware of changes so equipment can be properly cleaned.

- **Specific departmental leads:** Are you doing something that involves technology? Make sure to include the IT department. Something to do with a laboratory procedure? Reach out to laboratory services.

NOTE

This process is not just about getting approval. Take the time to know the stakeholders involved, and let them get to know you. It makes this process more enjoyable, and these connections you make now can be valuable in the future.

If you are a frontline staff member and need support in reaching out to these stakeholders, use your unit or departmental leaders to support you in this work. With their leadership experience come connections that will help move your project along.

Here's how the process can go, taking your idea to fruition:

- **Expect to trial your idea first.** Process improvement experts will want you to start small with a trial run. CHOP started with glucose testing bins in one or two patient rooms prior to committing to getting one placed in all 12 patient bed spaces. This would ensure that the process worked and saved money.

- **Obtain and gather the equipment you need.** Most hospital systems have a process in place for ordering supplies and equipment. You might think you can order your needed supplies from any internet site, but there are approved vendors and companies that your hospital prefers to order from. This type of information is very valuable and can only be gained by partnering with your individual leaders and managers who know the nuances of your specific hospital.

- **Cheerlead this work.** You have put in a lot of effort implementing this project—now be your own cheerleader. Educate the staff on the project. Utilize staff meetings, huddles, and any other opportunities you have to spread the word about this project.

- **Review the data and solicit feedback from the other staff members.** You can decide whether to adopt, adapt, or abandon the change, which is covered in Chapter 4. After installing the bins in three patient rooms, my nurse manager approved the use of the bin in each room throughout the unit. Things were up and running, and the bins became second nature. Staff were asking for more bins targeting different supplies because they loved having supplies at the bedside.

SEEING THE RESULTS

When you have implemented an idea, you next want to get results. You are probably curious if the efforts have the results you were expecting. Revisiting your data will allow you to see whether you have seen success in your project from a financial standpoint. Hopefully, you will see the results you desire. Celebrate and share those victories. In some instances, you will not see success. These projects are just as important to share with others.

There is a lot of learning that can happen from projects that were not successful. Other areas of the hospital may have had a similar idea. Sharing the roadblocks you encountered and the pitfalls can allow everyone to regroup and learn from your experience. Both failures and success are a learning experience.

In a few months, my unit saw a 98% reduction in the overall unit utilization of glucose testing strips, as shown in Figure 5.2.

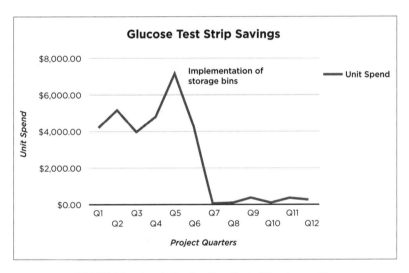

FIGURE 5.2 Graph showing the effect of the storage bins.

I could hardly contain my excitement and was so thrilled to share this work with both nursing-specific and hospital-wide presentations. We utilized these forums not only to highlight the success of our projects but to spread enthusiasm for the

CHOPtimize project. Keep these presentations fun, enthusiastic, and short. In a world of short attention spans and distractions, a fun and short presentation can help you keep your audience captivated.

PRIMARY AND SECONDARY GAINS

The primary gain is the fact that you helped contribute to the organization-wide cost-saving efforts. You should feel proud of the impact you have had in the reduction of usage and spend.

The financial savings does not have to be the only win. The personal and professional secondary gains you attain can far outweigh the financial gains. Here are just a few of the secondary gains you might experience:

- Share your story with others in the hospital. You can celebrate your success and encourage other units in their efforts.

- Present your story at national and international conferences. Figure 5.3 shows the CHOP group presenting at a conference. Submit an abstract for a poster or podium presentation.

- Write a book.

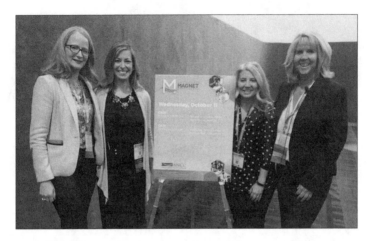

FIGURE 5.3 The CHOP team presenting at the 2017 ANCC Magnet
Conference.

The new process represents a true value—increasing the
quality of care while saving money. The storage units en-
sured continued compliance with keeping supplies labeled
and organized. The staff felt better knowing that, in a hypo-
glycemic event, all needed supplies to check and recheck a
blood glucose level were within reach.

6

FORWARD THINKING AND FINAL THOUGHTS

Mary Jo Gumbel, Supporting Practice & Management Chair for the Department of Nursing

WORDS &
CONCEPTS TO LEARN

Charge compliance

SuperUsers

Operations Managers

As we look back on this journey, we can see what tremendous progress we have made. We accomplished many targeted goals. Even though we found we were unsuccessful in some, we were able to learn valuable lessons, and most importantly, we laid out a path to continue this work well into our future. Financial stewardship is no longer a short-term goal on a hospital operating plan. It is no longer the sole responsibility of nurse executives. It is a standard of care for how nurses can help ensure the success of our institution and the top-notch care we give to our patients and families through a changing healthcare environment.

Financial stewardship has been embedded into the expectations of all that we do at CHOP, and it continues to challenge us all. CHOPtimize is a program embedded in clinical operations. It has become a way of doing things at this organization. The partnerships built with bedside staff through the Shared Governance model remain strong. Although we were able to witness a culture change with our initial work, continued passion and perseverance are necessary.

We want to also recognize how financial stewardship work can be easily transferred to a Professional Governance model. We firmly believe the ability to work collaboratively among interdisciplinary teams will generate even more ideas, process changes, and outcomes in promoting financial stewardship in your organization.

PROFESSIONAL GOVERNANCE

Professional Governance, previously known as Shared Governance, drives operational, professional, educational, and research processes for nursing practice . . . Councils are expected to integrate relevant professional and regulatory standards into their functions along with current research. (Genesis Health System, n.d., para. 1–2)

 NOTE

The CHOPtimize program was successful because of its system-wide approach. Creating a financial stewardship program around supply utilization and patient care practice that is given the same visibility as all other organizational goals was critical to its movement. Sharing successes and stories in group forums over the initial work allowed us to be open to improvement and create these new expectations. Transparency of data, dollars, and practice was critical to the work. Involving members of the organization across all departments where content experts were working with peers that didn't have direct interaction with supply utilization and patient care allowed us to push ourselves outside of our long-vetted practices. Empowering members of the team to lead individual projects with access to all data across all areas of the organization contributed to their buy-in and the spread of this program. Data trends, candid discussions, and looks in the garbage cans provided us with critical areas of focus. Transforming what began as an initiative into the norm is the key to sustaining this work. Creating an accepted standard of how we evaluate, use, and discuss what we do now seems normal and practical to our organization and will inevitably sustain long-term engagement and success.

The project that SPM has been highly invested in this past year was evaluating the practice of charging items. When frontline staff remove supplies from the locked supply cabinets, the item must be charged to the patient for whom it is being used. When looking at the hospital as a whole, there were opportunities identified for enhancing this process.

TALES FROM THE FRONT LINE

My name is Mary Jo Gumbel, and I am the current Supporting Practice & Management (SPM) Chair for the Department of Nursing, succeeding Megan by two terms. I became interested in this role not only by supporting the work that has been done in this council by the bedside nurses, but also because I truly look up to influencers and game changers in our profession. I feel strongly that when we come across obstacles in our line of work, we should not rely on management and higher-up executives to be the only problem solvers; rather, we should and must "be the change we want to see in the world," to quote Gandhi.

I'll be honest. I was not excited by this project when I started my role as chair. There was about a year's worth of work that went on behind the scenes by many smart people before I came into this role. I had a lot of catching up to do and needed to become an "early adopter" before bringing it to the unit chairs. There was a lot of high-level lingo, and I did not understand half of it. I had to help bring the work into terms that made sense to me as a bedside nurse before I could convince my unit chairs of its importance.

CREATING A NEW WORKFLOW

As we tackled this work, we quickly identified that most staff with access to the supply machine had never received formal training on the ideal process to charge for supplies removed. Training had only been offered to staff when the supply machines were installed many years prior.

We solved this by:

- Building a mandatory online module for all current staff.

- Creating a module for newly hired staff on how to remove items and charge for them, as well as review case scenarios for returning unused supplies, damaged supplies, and so on.

    This step was pivotal to engraining this work into nursing workflow. New frontline staff were now learning the process upon their orientation.

- Forming Charge Compliance Teams on each unit to maintain accountability. The teams consist of the SPM Unit Chair, *SuperUser* (specially trained staff member to troubleshoot and assist staff when using the supply machine), and Unit Managers who are ultimately responsible for their unit's compliance each month.

- Giving access to each unit chair to review their compliance each month (something we've never had access to before), and asking each chair to identify their supplies with the lowest levels of compliance.

This was not a smooth process at first, because there's never enough time away from everyday work responsibilities, and this work does not exactly flow into patient care.

To help jump-start the information sharing, I showcased each unit's compliance at the monthly SPM meeting, highlighted units that increased compliance from the previous month, and mentioned those units that had a significant decline. This was not to point blame at anyone but a way of sharing what was going well and what could be improved. Those units that showed great improvements were able to share best practices and help other units make positive changes for the following months. The units that were not doing as well were able to identify problems and share those. This was an important catalyst for many unit chairs to review processes on their own units.

After nearly all staff were trained using the modules, each unit assigned a Charge Compliance Team, and unit chairs became more invested in the work. We've asked each unit's Operations Manager to partner with the SPM Unit Chair to discuss charge compliance each month and discuss what those numbers mean. The Operations Managers have a unique role and are able to make sense of areas that we as bedside nurses may be missing, and vice versa. This has been a theme throughout the CHOPtimize journey: two very different roles working together and collaborating in ways they have not before.

CONTINUING EFFORTS

To ensure all parties are truly accountable to the new workflow, we implemented a monthly charge compliance data entry form that must be reviewed by the SPM Unit Chair, Operations Manager, and signed off by the unit's Nurse Manager. It is emailed directly to the Unit Chair each month and takes less than five minutes to complete. The form is then automatically sent to the managers for final review and signatures. This holds each party accountable and puts the bedside nurse in a vital role to guarantee that this work is sustained and not lost in the day-to-day craze that is the life of a nurse.

This fiscal year, the SPM Council will continue this important CHOPtimize work. We are brainstorming our next big initiative that includes an investigation into the ICU bedside carts and practices for disposing of supplies. This is an enormous cost to the hospital discovered only after a bedside nurse was asked, "Can you think of any ways that we are wasting money at the bedside?" Imagine that!

And now, thank you for taking the time to read about our journey. Good luck on yours.

REFERENCE

Genesis Health System. (n.d.). Professional governance. Retrieved from
https://www.genesishealth.com/careers/nursing/ghs/professional-
governance/

A

KEY DRIVER DIAGRAM (NONSALARY EXPENSE REDUCTION)

Nonsalary Expense Reduction: Key Driver Diagram

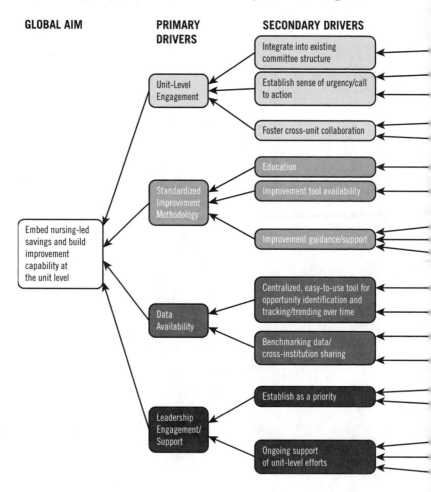

CHANGE CONCEPTS

Secure support to align with Nursing Shared Governance

Demonstrate financial concepts/forward-looking impacts (health rigor, etc.)

Senior leadership "elevator speeches"

Integrate sharing of accomplishments/lessons learned across units (local & organization-wide)

Tracking and sharing of unit progression through improvement framework

Administer staged introduction improvement framework phases/tools

Have standardized improvement tools readily available for units

Leadership and Improvement Department support

Align Nursing Shared Governance reps with unit-level quality and safety leaders for support

Align Nursing Shared Governance reps with similar organization-wide efforts (as appropriate)

Work with units/leaders to identify relevant breakdowns/access needed

Date tool training and ongoing support/refinement

Utilize Strategic Value Analysis listserv and benchmarking data available

Generate supply-specific SMART models (stories for success)

Establish targeted nonlabor reduction goals

Senior Leader "elevator speeches" to Nursing Shared Governance reps

Unit and organization-wide ongoing communication of savings effort importance and accomplishments

Assistance removing barriers encountered in pursuing savings opportunities

Local leaders engaged/demonstrate support/remove barriers

INDEX

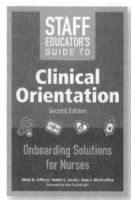
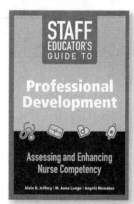
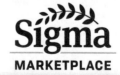

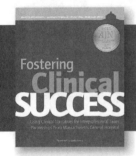 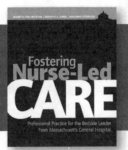 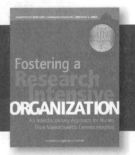
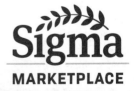

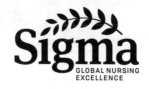

Sigma

GLOBAL NURSING EXCELLENCE

Sigma brings home more award:

CHECK OUT OUR 2018 *AMERICAN JOURNAL OF NURSING (AJ*
BOOK OF THE YEAR AWARDS

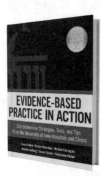

Evidence-Based Practice in Action

(9781940446936)

Second Place

**Education/Continuing Education/
Professional Development category**

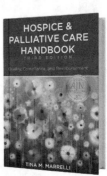

Hospice & Palliative Care Handbook
Third Edition

(9781945157455)

Second Place

Palliative Care and Hospice category

See Sigma's 2017 *AJN* Book of the Year Award recipients

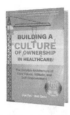

Building a Culture
of Ownership in
Healthcare

First Place

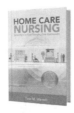

Home Care
Nursing

Second Place

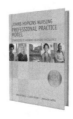

Johns Hopkins Nursing
Professional Practice
Model

Second Place

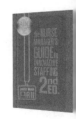

The Nurse Mana
Guide to Innova
Staffing, Second E

Third Place